Methods of
Cell Separation

Volume 3

BIOLOGICAL SEPARATIONS

Series Editor: **Nicholas Catsimpoolas**
Massachusetts Institute of Technology
Cambridge, Massachusetts

Methods of Protein Separation, Volume 1
Edited by Nicholas Catsimpoolas

Methods of Protein Separation, Volume 2
Edited by Nicholas Catsimpoolas

Biological and Biomedical Applications of Isoelectric Focusing
Edited by Nicholas Catsimpoolas and James Drysdale

Methods of Cell Separation, Volume 1
Edited by Nicholas Catsimpoolas

Methods of Cell Separation, Volume 2
Edited by Nicholas Catsimpoolas

Methods of Cell Separation, Volume 3
Edited by Nicholas Catsimpoolas

Methods of
Cell Separation

Volume 3

Edited by
Nicholas Catsimpoolas
Massachusetts Institute of Technology

Plenum Press · New York and London

Library of Congress Cataloging in Publication Data

Main entry under title:

Methods of cell separation.

  (Biological separations)
  Includes bibliographies and indexes.
  1. Cell separation. I. Catsimpoolas, Nicholas. II. Series. [DNLM: 1. Cell separa-
tion—Methods. WH25 M592]
QH585.M49   574.8'7'0724   77-11018
ISBN 0-306-40377-3 (v. 3)

© 1980 Plenum Press, New York
A Division of Plenum Publishing Corporation
227 West 17th Street, New York, N.Y. 10011

Printed in the United States of America

Contributors

Peter H. Bartels, *Optical Sciences Center, The University of Arizona, Tucson, Arizona*

Nicholas Catsimpoolas, *Biophysics Laboratory, Department of Nutrition and Food Science, Massachusetts Institute of Technology, Cambridge, Massachusetts*

Emil J. Freireich, *Department of Developmental Therapeutics, M.D. Anderson Hospital and Tumor Institute, The University of Texas System Cancer Center, Houston, Texas*

Jeane P. Hester, *Department of Developmental Therapeutics, M.D. Anderson Hospital and Tumor Institute, The University of Texas System Cancer Center, Houston, Texas*

Stephen M. Hunt, *Center for Blood Research, Boston, Massachusetts*

Robert M. Kellogg, *Biomedical Systems Division, IBM Corporation, Endicott, New York*

Paul L. Kronick, *Department of Physical and Life Sciences, Franklin Research Center, Philadelphia, Pennsylvania*

Fabian J. Lionetti, *Center for Blood Research, Boston, Massachusetts*

Kenneth B. McCredie, *Department of Developmental Therapeutics, M.D. Anderson Hospital and Tumor Institute, The University of Texas System Cancer Center, Houston, Texas*

Alfred Mulzet, *Biomedical Systems Division, IBM Corporation, Endicott, New York*

George B. Olson, *Department of Microbiology and Immunology, University of Arizona, Tucson, Arizona*

Chris D. Platsoucas, *Biophysics Laboratory, Department of Nutrition and Food Science, Massachusetts Institute of Technology, Cambridge, Massachusetts. Present address: Memorial Sloan-Kettering Cancer Center, New York, New York*

C. Robert Valeri, *Naval Blood Research Laboratory, Boston University Medical Center, Boston, Massachusetts*

Preface

Presently, the need for methods involving separation, identification, and characterization of different kinds of cells is amply realized among immunologists, hematologists, cell biologists, clinical pathologists, and cancer researchers. Unless cells exhibiting different functions and stages of differentiation are separated from one another, it will be exceedingly difficult to study some of the molecular mechanisms involved in cell recognition, specialization, interactions, cytotoxicity, and transformation. Clinical diagnosis of diseased states and use of isolated cells for therapeutic (e.g., immunotherapy) or survival (e.g, transfusion) purposes are some of the pressing areas where immediate practical benefits can be obtained by applying cell separation techniques. However, the development of such useful methods is still in its infancy. A number of good techniques exist based either on the physical or biological properties of the cells, and these have produced some valuable results. Still others are to be discovered. Therefore, the purpose of this open-ended treatise is to acquaint the reader with some of the basic principles, instrumentation, and procedures presently in practice at various laboratories around the world and to present some typical applications of each technique to particular biological problems. To this end, I was fortunate to obtain the contribution of certain leading scientists in the field of cell separation, people who in their pioneering work have struggled with the particular problems involved in separating living cells and who in some way have won. It is hoped that new workers with fresh ideas will join us in the near future to achieve further and much needed progress in this important area of biological research.

Nicholas Catsimpoolas

Cambridge, Massachusetts

Contents

Chapter 5

Biological Methods for the Separation of Lymphoid Cells

Chris D. Platsoucas and Nicholas Catsimpoolas

Computer Analysis of Lymphocyte Images

PETER H. BARTELS AND GEORGE B. OLSON

I. INTRODUCTION

Research on computer analysis of microscopic images of cells concentrates at this time on three major applications. These are the automated recognition of cells from the hematopoietic system, the analysis of epithelial cells and the study of lymphocyte populations. Of these, the first two are clearly related to the immediate needs of the clinical laboratory. White blood cell differential counts are carried out at a rate of more than 100 million per annum in the United States alone. Research and development here has progressed from the first feasibility studies accomplished in the 1960s by Preston (1961) and Preston (1962), Prewitt and Mendelsohn (1966), Ingram *et al.* (1968), Young (1969), and Bacus (1970) to the commercially available automated white blood cell differential counting devices. For the analysis of epithelial cells, the major effort has concentrated on the clinical cytology of the female reproductive tract (Wied *et al.*, 1976). Here, research toward the improvement of the diagnostic characterization of the material and extensive efforts to automate the prescreening for cervical cancer are underway. Also directed toward early detection and diagnosis of malignant disease, and particularly toward the extraction of prognostic clues, are research projects on image analysis of urothelial cells (Koss *et al.*, 1975, 1977a,b, 1978a; Bartels *et al.*, 1977c) and cells from the respiratory tract

PETER H. BARTELS ● Optical Sciences Center, The University of Arizona.   GEORGE B. OLSON ● Department of Microbiology and Immunology, University of Arizona, Tucson, Arizona 85721.

(Reale *et al.*, 1978; Wied *et al.*, 1979). The analysis of digitized images of lymphocytes at this time does not have such immediate clinical applications. Rather, image analysis has been applied as a research tool to (a) provide quantitative data for the assessment of the effects of biochemicals, immunobiologic agents, and ionizing radiation on lymphocyte populations (Bartels *et al.*, 1969a; Kiehn, 1972; McKee, 1975; Anderson, 1975a,b), (b) sharpen the discriminatory capabilities of the analytical computer software, and (c) to develop image analysis as a methodology (Bartels *et al.*, 1974).

A. Computable Image Information

One of the early and fascinating results of cell image analysis by the computer has been the realization that computation can extract information which the human eye does not perceive (Bartels *et al.*, 1972, 1974b; Bartels and Wied, 1975a; Wied *et al.*, 1968). Such information is contained in the distribution pattern of the nuclear chromatin. For example, the value of the conditional probability with which a chromatin granule of a certain optical density (OD) occurs at a given location in the nucleus—provided that a granule of another OD had been observed at a certain other location—is not consciously perceived. Human visual perception appears to be insensitive to higher-order statistical textures (Julesz, 1962, 1975; Julesz *et al.*, 1973). Mutual dependencies between numerical values in the digitized cell image, particularly when an extended local neighborhood is considered, are not perceived to a degree that would allow small differences to be clearly recognized. Furthermore, beyond the mutual dependencies of the OD values in the digitized image, the human visual sense provides no clues to the descriptive statistics of the underlying mutual dependence scheme. For example, if one described the mutual dependence by a multivariate process, visual observation will not provide an estimate for the value of a coefficient of one of the eigenvectors of that process. "Computable image information" of this kind has up to now never been used for diagnostic decision making, or even the objective characterization of cell images. The discriminatory power of computation may thus be used to expand our ability to perceive small differences (Bartels and Subach, 1976). Computable image information may not only be used to describe the chromatin distribution pattern of cells of known type in objective, numerical terms. In addition, computed image information may be used to detect differences between cells which appear identical to the eye and to detect minute and early changes in cells.

B. Chromatin Distribution Patterns

The chromatin distribution pattern in a cell nucleus is determined by (a) the number and size distribution of the chromatin granules, (b) their staining density, and (c) their spatial arrangement. The chromatin may be described as coarse or fine in granularity as well as uniformly distributed or as aggregated, and one may assess the tendency of the chromatin to concentrate near the nuclear membrane or the center of the nucleus. For cells of a given type or in a given physiologic state, the chromatin distribution pattern is surprisingly consistent and provides for highly reproducible features. Yet, features derived from the chromatin distribution pattern enable one to detect very early responses of a cell to changes in (a) physiologic conditions or (b) to external influences such as ionizing radiation, virus infections, immunologically active agents, and pharmaceutical and toxic substances. Research efforts toward the objective characterization of nuclear chromatin distribution patterns have addressed two major problems. The first is the methodology of introducing a mensuration to what has so far been a strictly subjective procedure; that is, the visual microscopic examination of cells by a cytologist. How can one characterize such chromatin distribution patterns and what measures or features could one define? How can one compute and evaluate these features? How may one apply them for an objective classification or description of a response or a trend? The second problem bears reference to the biologic meaning of these measures. How can one interpret the measures themselves or the observed changes in terms of biologic processes? Of these two problems, the first becomes a prerequisite for a study of the second. The two problems may be addressed independently but it is clear that they are closely related. One can establish a highly successful automated classification procedure for different cell types, e.g., normal and malignant cells. The classifier may use features which consistently render excellent discrimination. To accomplish this, one does not have to have any insight into the biologic reasons as to why these features assume certain values in malignant cells and markedly different values in normal cells. On the other hand, a more satisfactory situation exists whenever a known biologic process can be closely correlated with the value distribution for a given feature and a biologic interpretation is possible. Under these conditions one can measure a biologic response directly. It is well known that the degree of condensation of the nuclear chromatin as heterochromatin or euchromatin reflects different levels of functional activity. Heterochromatin is associated with a lower level of genetic activity. The relationship between heterochromatin and euchromatin and the functional state of cells was explored in several studies by

Kiefer and Sandritter (Sandritter *et al.*, 1967; Sandritter and Kiefer, 1970; Kiefer *et al.*, 1971, 1973, 1974). Increasing differentiation or maturation leads to larger proportions of the nuclear chromatin assuming a condensed form. The ratio of heterochromatin to euchromatin is well defined and varies only within narrow tolerances in cells of a given cell type and in a given physiologic state. Sandritter *et al.* (1967) determined the proportion of heterochromatin in peripheral lymphocytes as 80% whereas lymphoblasts contain 40–60% heterochromatin. Dedifferentiating cells are characterized by a predominance of euchromatic material. The increase in heterochromatin and the loss of genetic information has been described as a pathogenic principle by Sandritter and others (Harbers and Sandritter, 1968; Harbers *et al.*, 1968). Marked changes in the ratio of heterochromatin to euchromatin were observed in transforming lymphocytes (Bartels *et al.*, 1969; Rowinski *et al.*, 1972). For a survey of research efforts aimed at the methodology of cell-image analysis, the reader is referred to the monographs by Wied *et al.* (1970a, 1976), to the proceedings of the First Life Sciences Conference at Los Alamos (Richmond *et al.*, 1975), and to the literature survey given by Preston (1976) and Prewitt (1972). Papers reporting descriptions of cell image features which are suitable for an assessment of the chromatin distribution pattern or of the methodology of classification by supervised learning and unsupervised learning procedures are referenced in this text.

II. SELECTION OF EQUIPMENT

The biomedical researcher who wishes to install an image-analysis facility has to make a number of decisions about the configuration of the system and about specific components. At this stage of the planning process it is very worthwhile to discuss one's plans with researchers who are now operating such facilities, and with personnel from one's own institution to determine what support in digital electronics design, engineering, and computer programming is locally available. One of the major systems components is an optical microscope photometer.

A. The Microscope Photometer

If the system is intended primarily for the study of lymphocytes, a microscope photometer with scanning stage and a photomultiplier attachment is an excellent choice. Lymphocytes are comparatively small cells and scan field sizes from 20 × 20 to 60 × 60 bracket the range for most applications. A spatial sampling interval of 0.5 μm has been found adequate in our studies (Wied *et al.*, 1970a; Bartels and Wied, 1975b); if a sampling interval of 0.25 μm is considered necessary, this is still manageable. The optical microscope employed in microphotometry should be designed for high mechanical stability, especially if the photometer attachment is attached directly to the microscope stand. Most research microscopes follow a modular design principle. This allows for great versatility and is a valid design principle. In microphotometry, however, it has proven to pose serious problems. Every attachment, every adapter ring, every extra observation port becomes a potential source of stray light. The user is well advised to check all such connections and to tape them carefully. In the recording of cell images, use of a 100× oil immersion objective is common. The condenser is usually a 0.30 N.A. microscope objective with an extra long working distance. If a condenser system with an adjustable aperture stop is provided, it is advisable to lock its position permanently to assure reproducibility of results. The condenser centering mounts provided by commercial optical companies are totally inadequate for microphotometry. They do not permit the required precise position control, the control knobs are small, and in several models are all but inaccessible. Their threading is too coarse to allow for smooth and definitive control, and they tend not to hold the condenser in the precisely centered position. In actual use, the operator may have to adjust the condenser centration literally hundreds of times. The user of a scanning microscope photometer may find it necessary to design his own condenser-centering mount. A fixed field stop, restricting the illuminated field in the object plane to an area approximately 5 μm in diameter, is essential to keep stray light low. This field stop should be easily removable so that the operator may see the whole field of view when searching for cells or mapping cell locations. The insertion of the field stop before measurement requires a high degree of positional reproducibility. Its mount should be centerable, with an adequate range. In object-plane scanning microphotometers, as described, the delineation of the actually measured spot is accomplished by means of a small measuring stop mounted in an intermediary image plane. Its area corresponds to the chosen spot size, e.g., 0.5×0.5 μm^2 in the object plane. Round and square measuring apertures are employed: results are not directly comparable since the convolution of the image of the corresponding object area by the two types of aperture is different. Adjustable apertures carry the constant risk of change in setting and are not desirable. It is important that the operator can conveniently make frequent checks of the coincidence of the measuring aperture and its position target in the ocular by use of a crosshair or small engraved circle. If an adjustment is needed, this should be possible over a reasonable range with smooth but tightly threaded controls. Scanning stages typically are driven by stepping motors. There are manufacturers who offer scanning stages with a 2×2 cm range, with 0.5-μm increments and 200 steps/s. Other manufacturers offer dual stages; a coarse stage with an incremental step of 10 μm spanning a wide range and a 0.5μm-increment stage with a 200 × 200 μm range. The fine stage is mounted on top of the coarse stage. Both arrangements make workable systems but both also pose problems.

The wide-range 0.5-μm-increment stages have frequently been found to suffer from resonance effects when run at full design speed. Scan lines may be out of register, may not have formed rectangular scan fields, or may have skipped points. The dual stage arrangement requires software which will keep track of how many steps were taken in what direction on both the coarse and the fine stage. As a rule, it is not true that twenty 0.5-μm steps taken with the fine stage correspond precisely to a single 10-μm step. Failure to keep count will let the computer get hopelessly lost and unable to relocate mapped objects. A newer scanning stage capable of 10,000 Hz, with 0.25-μm increments and a continuous driven motor, is also available. At the present time, the manufacturer does not supply a software system for its operation.

In recent years the value of spectral information has been appreciated more and more. Photomultiplier attachments with three photomultiplier tubes and a set of dichroic beam splitters appear to be the method of choice to record images in three wavelength bands so that the three images are in fixed registration. One may transfer the three images simultaneously to three A/D converters and sample them sequentially by the data-acquisition software. One may also use a multiplexer and offer the images sequentially to a single A/D converter. The latter operation is more time consuming but more economical. For each photomultiplier tube, a separate operational amplifier has to be provided so that each channel can be adjusted to 100% transmission in the free background. Independent dark current controls are also needed. It is customary to digitize the analog photo signal to 8 bits. This corresponds to a byte, or half a word of the usual 16-bit computer word. Eight bits can represent 256 gray levels. Few microspectrophoto- meters do indeed reach such photometric precision. For a very few custom- built instruments, the signal to noise ratio is better than 200:1. For most commercial instruments the actual signal to noise ratio varies from 100:1 to 60:1. This corresponds to 1.0–1.5% photometric noise and a precision of from 7 to 6 bits. Results obtained on a given microphotometer are highly reproducible. However, there are substantive differences in the contrast transfer function of different models of microphotometers made by differ- ent manufacturers and even within the same company. Qualitative results, such as the kind of features contributing to a discrimination, tend to agree between data recorded on a variety of different instruments. Quantita- tively, distinctively different decision rules and feature values are found.

With the increasing use of this methodology, introduction of an industry standard should receive serious consideration.

B. Interface

The microscope and its photometric accessories are linked to the computer by an interface. There are two major functions involved in the control of the scanning microphotometer by the computer. These are the collection of image data from the photometer and the operation of the scanning stage. These two must be rigidly coordinated. A typical sequence of operations during data recording is as follows. The operator looks through the microscope and searches for a cell to be scanned. For this, the stage is controlled manually by means of a joystick. The computer keeps track of the stage's x and y positions. Once a cell is found, the operator presses a ''store'' button on the interface and the computer stores the x,y coordinates in a location map on a disc file. The operator is now free to search for the next cell. The mapping program is particularly useful when an expert is required to identify the cells to be measured. The program allows the specialist to designate a large number of cells for measurement within a relatively short time. The measurements themselves may then be taken by a technician. The search for cells is frequently conducted so that cell selection is randomized. Even before the first cell is located, the operator uses the joystick to circumscribe the area on the slide where cells are found. This boundary is stored by the computer. A program then generates a pair of random numbers denoting an x and a y coordinate. The generated stage position is checked against the stored boundary. If it falls inside the area containing cells, the stepping motors drive the stage to that location. The cell nearest to the crosshair center in the field of view is chosen for measurement. If the randomly generated stage position falls outside the boundary, a new coordinate pair is generated automatically. Another method for mapping cells on a microscope slide and for the exchange of microscope slides between different institutions employs the use of a glass stage micrometer. With this procedure, it is possible to locate a cell within an accuracy of one micron.

After a set of cells has been mapped, the computer recalls the coordinates of the first cell. The operator enters the number of steps per scan line and the number of scan lines. He positions the scanning stage at the upper left-hand corner of the intended scan field and makes a test scan. The test scan merely drives the stage around the periphery of the outlined scan field. It shows the operator whether the cell is completely enclosed by the area. If no correction is needed, the light transmission is corrected to zero OD. This may be accomplished by several methods. One method is to set the value of the starting background point to zero OD. A second method is to determine the mean value of the light points of one scan line and equate this to zero OD. A third method is to scan the entire scan, checking to be sure all values are within the 256 gray levels, and by use of a software program determine that the maximum values of the first peak of the histogram are declared to be zero OD. Scanning is then initiated.

Scanning proceeds in discrete incremental steps. When the stage has arrived at a point, the program waits for a specified amount of time to allow for settling of mechanical vibrations. The analog signal from the photomultiplier tube, i.e., the photocurrent, is then sent to the A/D converter, sampled, and averaged a number of times. If more than one wavelength is recorded, this is done for all channels. Once the value is digitized, a "ready" signal is issued. The stepping motor takes an incremental step. The step counters are updated. A determination is made to ascertain whether the next scan line has to be started. When the scan is completed, the stage is driven back to the starting point. At this time, the operator is offered the option to discard the recorded scan field and to rescan it. If the scan is accepted, the program assigns a name to the cell image. An ID number and pertinent header information for the data file, such as wavelength, spatial resolution, name of the operator, and date, are automatically entered. The map file is updated and the cell is identified as already scanned. The operator is informed how many cells are still to be scanned. For the use of the manual joystick, it is desirable to have a nonlinear response built into the software. When the joystick is held at a large deflection, the stage should run fast. When one wants an exact positioning, the stepping motors should step very slowly.

It is essential to have some sort of visual display so that the scan field can be edited while the original cell is still in the field of view. "Editing" means the elimination of data points that fall into the scan field but are not part of the cell. Rather, they may be due to debris, uneven background due to staining or portions of other cells. For the editing, one may use an interactive program. One may display a cursor which can be driven by the joystick. This cursor can then be used to draw an outline. Everything outside that outline is discarded. One may also use a cursor box where a small frame is displayed and moved around by the joystick. The cursor box is used much like a vacuum cleaner: every point that falls into the cursor box is automatically eliminated.

The editing may be done entirely by software. The display then merely shows the results, which one may accept or reject. In the latter case the algorithm will request the entering of new parameters, such as a new boundary threshold. We have found it practical never to discard any of the originally recorded data points. Edited points are merely set to negative values. They can thus always be restored.

C. Computer

The ideal situation exists when the computer is reserved exclusively for the cell-image-analysis project. To take full advantage of analytical software that is available for cell image analysis, a moderate-size computer is required. A machine with at least 64K core memory is highly desirable. The TICAS 11/45 software runs on an 88K PDP 11/45, under RXS 11 D, which unfortunately requires a high overhead in core just for the operating system. All tasks of the TICAS 11/45 package are overlaid to fit into the 32K task size; the restriction is imposed by the 16-bit word length of the PDP 11/45. The newer computers offer 32-bit word length and this is preferable. A 32-bit word offers the advantage of efficient storage of cell images recorded at three different wavelengths with 8 bits, or 256 gray levels for each image and the possibility of forming transformed or composite images in the remaining 8 bits.

It is not, as a rule, a satisfactory solution when the microscope photometer is interfaced to a laboratory computer which is utilized and owned by someone else. Data acquisition in cell image analysis is time consuming. It may occupy the computer for several hours each day. Even when the software allows for several simultaneous users, e.g., by "time slicing," mutual dissatisfaction may develop. Certain functions of the operating system have priorities which disrupt everything else. Situations are not infrequent where either party may sit for minutes at a time just waiting to be able to continue his work while the system is racing back and forth in an attempt to serve all demands, but with steeply decreasing efficiency. If a laboratory computer has to be shared, the only practical solution is to have the microscope photometer and the image data acquisition controlled by a microprocessor, such as, for example, a DEC* LSI 11 system. In this way interaction with the main computer is reduced and can be coordinated by the operating system for high efficiency. Control of the microscope photometer by a microprocessor is a very desirable configuration in any case, even when a dedicated computer is available. Image data acquisition may then proceed without interfering with program development and data analysis.

One may provide for a general interface to control the microscope photometer and use interface cards supplied by the computer manufacturer. One may also employ modules such as the DEC Lab peripheral system which has a number of A/D converters and several channels to drive peripherals.

A large disc is essential. A disc with 10 megawords is the very mini-

* Digital Equipment Corporation, Maynard, Massachusetts.

mum, but discs with 80–300 megawords are available at not greatly increased cost. It is important to realize that it is foolhardy to operate such a system without the ability to make frequent system backups. For this, either a second disc drive is needed—and for the large discs this is almost the only practically feasible solution—or one has to have a magnetic tape drive. For the tape drive the trend is toward 9-track tapes. A system backup for a 10-megaword disc may require several tapes and may take up to three hours. The tapes used to generate the updated weekly backup should be discarded after six months of use since frequent reading and writing leads to the occasional loss of bits and a gradual corruption of the system.

A most valuable addition to any laboratory computer used for image processing and analysis is an array processor. Array processors provide for extremely high-speed computing; their architecture is designed to take full advantage of the structure of the data. When the data to be processed are in the form of an array, such as a digitized image or a list of feature values, the design of array processors allows for an increase of computation speed by a factor of about one hundred. The greater efficiency in processing of data arrays utilizes "parallel processing" and "pipelining." This is best explained by an example. Multiplying two floating-point numbers typically involves three steps. First the fractions are multiplied, then the exponents are added, and finally the result is normalized and rounded. These three steps are carried out in sequence, i.e., while the second step is taken, the hardware for the first and the third step waits idle. In pipelining, as soon as the first step is completed for the first element of the array, and the hardware is free, the first step for the second element is taken, concurrently with step two for the first element. When step three is taken for the first element, step two is taken for the second element, and step one for the third element—all concurrently. Once the pipeline is full, a result is obtained at every step and not only at every third step as in conventional arithmetic processors. There are floating-point array processors available now which can deliver 12,000,000 floating-point computations per second.

By providing in the hardware architecture of the processor multiple instruction and data paths, a high degree of parallelism can be achieved. For example, processing may call for (a) incrementing a data address, (b) retrieving the data from that address, (c) performing an arithmetic operation of that value, (d) possibly updating a loop counter, and (e) determining whether the loop is completed. All of these are done in sequence and by separate instructions in a conventional processor. In an array processor this entire set of instructions may be carried out in parallel and by a single instruction. Array processors appear to be ideally suited for employment in a systems configuration for the preprocessing of cell images, feature extraction, and for the processing of feature lists and matrices.

Next on the list of peripherals is an interactive display. Full color visual graphic displays offer several advantages. The programmer is aided in the examination of the mode of action of certain algorithms, e.g., of nuclear boundary finding routines or of scene segmentation algorithms. The option to display singly or a combination of images recorded at different wavelengths helps in the utilization of spectral information for feature design. Artificial color encoding of certain features permits display of the topographic distribution of their values: this allows a visualization, for example, of the spatial patterns of features based on first-order statistics and the formulation of new features based on higher-order statistics. The full color capability furthermore permits clinical researchers to inspect the data base directly.

D. Photomicrography and Video-Recording

For certain studies it is almost mandatory that a color photomicro-graphic record of the original cell images be kept for later visual confirmation, diagnostic appraisal, or reassessment. With the availability of automated 35-mm photomicrographic cameras the recording of these images is made much easier and reliable. Yet it still adds a considerable amount of time to the recording of each cell image. Much more serious, however, is the storage and display problem. It is not unusual to have 20,000 cell images recorded in a given study.

Videotape recording offers considerable advantage over 35-mm photography for mass storage. The recorder should have facilities for single frame recording and retrieval; a character generator is used to provide identification for the image or to enter results from visual and/or computer assessment.

III. COMPUTER PROGRAMS

The essence of the power of computerized cell image analysis rests with the capabilities of the analytical software. Every installation builds up a collection of programs which evolve, sometimes over many years, into a comprehensive analytical system. There are software systems which have absorbed up to 100 man-years of programming efforts. These program systems have cost more than the original combined purchase price of the microscope photometer and the computer. They are a most valuable asset.

A. Design Considerations

Developing such an image-analytical-program package is a major endeavor. It is worthwhile to consider some of the rationale that went into the development of the TICAS program package and the experiences gained there. One of the prime considerations in the design of this program system was ease of use for the biomedical researcher. There should never be a situation where the user confronts the terminal, the computer is waiting for some input but the user either does not know what is expected of him, or he cannot remember what input a certain program at that particular point requires. The system should at all times display on the CRT options, questions, or instructions in full plain English text. The system should specify which answers are valid options. The user should not have to remember any computer operating system commands. The user should not have to remember program names nor feature names. The user should at all times be able to request the display of HELP information. The user should not have to remember which kinds of files are available: he should merely have to decide from a selection list which files he wants to use.

An important consideration is ease of maintenance of the program package. This is closely related to the availability of documentation. In the TICAS 11/45 package, FORTRAN is used throughout. The only exception are short subroutines which are device drivers. These are of necessity written in assembler language. It is true that there are image processing tasks that would benefit greatly from execution by some specialized language. However, strict adherence to FORTRAN has enabled us over twelve years to maintain, update, and document our extensive program library. It is not necessary to hire specialized programmers. New personnel become quickly familiar with existing programs, are able to change them, and document the changes. The TICAS 11/45 program package as a whole, or in parts, has been transferred to a substantial number of other computer installations with a minimum of difficulties. These involved primarily three issues.

First, when any program in FORTRAN or in any other language, is transferred to another computer, one should check whether program parameters, such as, for example, in optimization routines the smallest increment which is considered an improvement, are compatible with the numerical precision offered by the word length of the computer.

Second, even though the programs handling and staging the data, i.e., forming, retrieving, merging, and dividing feature files are written in FORTRAN, they do rely on certain capabilities of the RSX 11 D operating system. Other computer systems may have different ways of setting up files.

Third, the assembler subroutines to drive the peripherals must be rewritten.

The user should receive adequate help during the interactive use of the system. HELP displays are required at several levels. When different programs are offered as options, there is a need to explain what they do. The program name is usually not sufficiently explanatory. After the user has selected a program, he needs to be informed about logistic requirements, such as "Your data must be on disc 1," and about restrictions, such as "This program accepts a maximum of 600 data points." There are programs which require the output from another program. The user must be reminded to run the other program first.

It is helpful to have results interpreted. Most computer programs provide quite a bit of printed output. Much of this is needed for a later in-depth look at the data, as background information, or as a basis for further data extraction. The most important results though are usually just a few values, rarely more than five to ten. The user who is familiar with the programs and the problem knows where to look for these particular values and how to interpret them. The beginner should be directed, by the system, to these key results and instructed as to what their significance is. This can be done with a short narrative. For example, let it be assumed that a table of variables and their correlations with a certain discriminant function is printed out. It then helps to say: Such and such variables have the highest correlation with the discriminant function: they make the most important contribution to the separation of the data sets. Format compatibility is an important issue. All data files are written in a standardized format. Each and every program uses that format for its input and output. In this fashion the results from any program are acceptable as input data for any other program. "Results" here are to be understood in a wide sense. The results may be (a) the values of a set of features to be filed as a feature file; (b) the probability that a given feature is found for a cell from a given cell category: these probabilities are filed in feature files for potential use as a descriptive, probabilistically defined feature; (c) the assignment to a subset of cells by an unsupervised learning algorithm: the cluster assignment is filed in the same format as a feature so that all items assigned to a given cluster can be retrieved on the basis of that property; and (d) an assignment by a supervised learning and classification algorithm: filing group membership in feature format allows one to retrieve all cells correctly classified or misclassified.

When a substantial number of analytical programs are available, it is difficult to remember all of them and even more difficult to remember their names and their requirements. In order to offer the user a fully transparent system with an immediate display of all available programs and without the need to use system commands, the TICAS 11/45 package employs a monitor program. This program offers all analytical programs arranged in a hierarchy. The user only has to choose options and is guided through any sequence of tasks that his problem may require. The monitor program automatically opens and closes files. It takes the user back to the monitor program once an analytical program has been completed. It can accommodate as many analytical programs as the number of different tasks that the computer can handle; this can be set to a very substantive number at the time the computer operating system is set up, i.e., at "system generation" time. All that is required to add a new program is that it be debugged, compiled, entered and installed as a task, that the option frame be updated, and the text on the HELP frame be entered.

B. Data Staging and File Handling

All of the analytical programs may thus be offered in an easily understood and manageable form under control of the monitor program. The user has no need to learn the system commands. The handling of files, i.e., data storage and retrieval, requires extensive software. This is supplied by the manufacturer of the computer and offered as part of the operating system. Unfortunately, this requires that the user become thoroughly familiar with the system's commands, and, in our experience, this has led to problems. The data-handling software, such as the peripheral interchange program package PIP of the DEC, cannot be called from a FORTRAN program. Thus, the user has to leave the monitor program to be able to handle files. We found it worthwhile to get assistance from the DEC software specialists who modified our operating system so that we can call PIP from any FORTRAN program. The user is then finally freed from the need to remember the operating system commands. In practical work in image analysis, one will find that a surprising amount of data handling is routinely required. There is the constant need to establish, to eliminate, to rename, to merge, or to subdivide files. One may wish to select items sequentially or at random. Furthermore, one may wish to retrieve certain items from one or several different files, to eliminate certain items from a file or to rename individual items. There is also a need to transfer files from one storage device to another, e.g., from tape to disc or from one disc to another, and to store data on tape.

A computer with an operating system which is not file-oriented, but can retrieve data only on a "block" basis, is quite unsuitable for cell image analysis work. Also, it is highly desirable to be able to access data not only by name but also by value. For example, the computer will, by means of its system software, readily retrieve any data file once the file name is specified. It is a different matter when from a given file, or collection of files, one wants to retrieve all cells which have a certain property. For example, one may wish to retrieve all T cells which have a nuclear area larger than a certain threshold. There are elegant, but unfortunately, also costly solutions to this problem. One may purchase and install special data-management software. Even the better program packages, however, demand a certain rigidity with respect to the number of features per cell that will be computed or how many spectral images one wishes to store. It is not that the software could not accommodate any change. It is just that any change requires conversion of the entire data base, and this can be cumbersome. To retrieve all cells with a nuclear area beyond a certain size, the management software will examine each cell data file, determine whether or not the value for the nuclear area falls into the desired range, and place the cell ID into an output file, if this is the case.

On the PDP 11/45 we elected to develop a very flexible but not quite as elegant method which has proven itself to be eminently practical. Instead of filing each digitized cell image and its features in sequence in a common file, the 11/45 package creates separate feature files. Each group of features has a common file extension, e.g., the relative frequencies of OD values have a file extension; in the FORTRAN code of the PDP 11 computers, this would be denoted by ".HST." Each extension holds up to 25 features. One can then retrieve feature values directly without going to each cell-image file. By using an interactive display, a feature-value distribution can be displayed. The user sets a cursor and all cells with a feature value in a certain range of values are put into a subfile. This is faster than the method described above. The practical use is demonstrated in Fig. 1. One displays a feature and notices a marked bimodality. One can now readily form two

```
FEATURE NAME : SDMF1

RANGE   PERCENT TOTAL

-1.800    1.19 (   3)  I*****
-1.600    1.59 (   4)  I******
-1.400    9.13 (  23)  I***********************************
-1.200   13.10 (  33)  I***************************************************
-1.000    9.13 (  23)  I***********************************
-0.800    7.14 (  18)  I***************************
-0.600    3.97 (  10)  I***************
-0.400    3.17 (   8)  I*************
-0.200    0.79 (   2)  I***
 0.000    1.98 (   5)  I*********
 0.200    2.78 (   7)  I************
 0.400    3.17 (   8)  I**************
 0.600   13.10 (  33)  I***************************************************
 0.800    8.73 (  22)  I*********************************
 1.000    7.54 (  19)  I*****************************
 1.200    8.73 (  22)  I*********************************
 1.400    3.97 (  10)  I*****************
 1.600    0.40 (   1)  I*
 1.800    0.40 (   1)  I*
 2.000    0.00 (   0)  I

WANT TO CREATE SUB-FILE : N
```

FIGURE 1. Computer printout of a distribution of a feature value showing the bimodal distribution of the lymphocytes into two modes with approximate mean values of -1.20 and $+0.8$.

subfiles for further analysis. The example shown is for the distribution of values of a discriminant function. The user can specify a name for the subfile and transfer all cell IDs whose feature values for the displayed feature fall into the specified range into the subfile. For this subfile then, the values of all other features can be obtained quickly. However, data-management software can very quickly retrieve data defined by Boolean expressions, e.g., retrieve all cells where the nuclear area is between two given values and which have an average staining density above a given threshold, but only if the maximum OD in the red spectral region is higher than that in the blue spectral region. The 11/45 software has to do this sort of retrieval successively, which is possible, but not very elegant.

IV. ANALYTICAL TASKS

The practical problems encountered in cell image analysis fall into a number of well defined analytical situations.

First, there are discrimination and classification tasks (Fukunaga, 1972). A cell image is to be assigned to one of several known types of cells. Decision rules for such assignments are to be determined. For example, an unknown cell image is to be classified as a B cell or a T cell, or an unknown cell image is to be classified as virus-infected or not infected. Furthermore, the discrimination may involve more than two cell categories. A cell image may then be classified according to a simultaneous classification strategy or the classification sequence may follow a hierarchy of decision nodes (Taylor et al., 1974, 1978a; Kulkarni and Kanal, 1976). For example, consider the possibility that a cell image is either a B cell, a T cell, or a monocyte. The simultaneous decision rule would typically decide: this cell is, for example, a monocyte. A hierarchic decision sequence may decide at the first decision node: this cell is not a B cell, therefore it is either a T cell or a monocyte. At the second decision node, the decision that it is a monocyte would be made.

Second, there are tasks which explore the homogeneity of a set of cell images. Visual examination cannot always distinguish cell images, but the structure of the extracted cell image features may reveal the existence of modes or subsets of cells with statistically significantly different patterns of their nuclear chromatin distribution (Bartels et al., 1974c). Visual confirmation becomes effective when the inhomogeneity of a set of cell images expresses itself in a clearly detectable bimodality in the distribution of one or more of the recorded cell image features. However, the bimodality or the multimodality may not be obvious and may require the simultaneous consideration of perhaps a dozen variables. Computer algorithms must then be used to search for and detect these modes (Anderberg, 1973; Hartigan, 1975).

Third, there are trend analyses. For example, experimental animals or cells from tissue cultures are exposed to a treatment. The treatment may consist of a single exposure or be administered in multiple sequential exposures. In either case, the subsequent changes and response of the affected cell populations are studied as a function of time. The objectives are to answer such questions as: (a) Does the treatment cause a measureable effect? (b) Which cell image properties or combinations of cell image properties lend themselves as good indicators of the response? (c) What is the smallest effect that can be detected and statistically secured? (d) How can the effect and the trendal changes which it causes be quantitated and defined? (e) Does the entire exposed cell population respond in a like manner or are there subsets of cells which are less affected?

The analytical software consists of a number of modules which can be combined and rearranged to meet the requirements of each of these tasks. The program modules are for:

1. Feature extraction and establishment of feature files
2. Feature evaluation and selection
3. Supervised learning and classification
4. Nonsupervised learning and clustering
5. Statistical analysis

A classification task typically requires only the feature extraction, feature evaluation, and classification program modules. Supervised learning, cell discrimination, and classification require the following program module sequence:

1. Feature extraction
2. Feature evaluation
3. Feature selection
4. Supervised learning, derivation of a classification rule
5. Test of the classification rule by classification programs

The nonsupervised learning and homogeneity testing tasks usually employ program modules in a more complicated combination. Feature extraction is followed by a feature evaluation and selection; but this is possible only for a small number of features at one time because of the memory-core requirements demanded by most unsupervised learning algorithms. After a clustering algorithm has been run, the subsets of cells assigned to different clusters are tested for statistical differences (Beale, 1969). The subsets are then submitted to a supervised learning algorithm. These programs permit an effective identification of further features which may be useful to detect these subsets. The best discriminating features are then selected and resubmitted to the clustering algorithm and statistical testing for significance of differences. A typical program module sequence is:

1. Feature extraction
2. Feature selection: first subset of features, clustering algorithm
3. Multivariate significance test of partitioning; if necessary, it will go through several subsets of features until a valid partitioning of clusters is obtained
4. Submission of clusters to supervised learning algorithm to be used as training sets for feature selection
5. Selection of best features
6. Submission to unsupervised learning algorithm
7. Multivariate significance test

The response and trend analyses also involve complicated sequencing of program modules. If an untreated control group of cells and a group of cells representing maximum exposure are available, feature evaluation may be done using these two groups of cells as prototypes. It is advisable, however, to examine both the control and the end stage groups of cells first for homogeneity. If a cell group is found to be homogeneous, or to have responded homogeneously, it is accepted as such. If, however, inhomogeneities are found in either cell sample, their response has to be followed separately. This will usually require an examination of the subpopulations, their proportions, and their properties for a number of intermediate exposures. Using the classification rules derived above, one may proceed, when intermediate sets of observations are available, to classify cells in the intermediate treatment sets as being affected or not affected. One may also test for homogeneity in each of the intermediate treatment sets and compare the cell images assigned to different modes to control cells. All cell images indistinguishable from control cells are then classified as "not affected" and merged into a file of "normal cells." All affected cells, assigned to different modes by the clustering algorithms, are analyzed for mean feature values and trends as a function of treatment duration or intensity.

Experiments of this kind can lead to very complicated changes in data sets as a function of time. For example, in carcinogenesis experiments, application of a carcinogen may lead to an immediate toxic reaction which persists only for a limited length of time. After this, cells may begin to return to a more normal state. Finally, a certain percentage of cells have returned to the normal state, and the rest may progress to cytologic conditions which may be termed premalignant or malignant. Analysis of such data sets would involve clusters in feature space which persist only during certain periods of time, then disappear, to be replaced by other clusters. As a rule, the detection of subsets of cells undergoing different responses requires different feature spaces for each subset. Feature selection, therefore, has to be optimized for each point in time.

In the following text, the application of different analytical programs is demonstrated with a number of practical examples. In the TICAS 11/45 software package the program modules for feature extraction, selection, supervised learning and unsupervised learning, and classification may be applied to three different levels of image analysis (Bartels and Wied, 1977). The first level is concerned with image points. The second level involves individual cell images, and the third level addresses the analysis of whole cell populations and their representation by profiles.

At the first level, the reliable tracking of a nuclear boundary, for example, may require the identification of cell image points which are ''boundary points.'' A boundary point has distinctive properties. Its immediate neighbors can be expected, for example, to differ greatly in their optical density. One may extract information describing the local neighborhood relationships for each image point and form an ''image-point feature vector.'' Then, one may use the feature evaluation, selection, and classification programs to assign every point in the cell image into one of three classes: inside the nucleus, outside the nucleus, and boundary point. The location file of all points assigned to the class of boundary points is then used to trace the nuclear boundary. It is stored in the form of a chain code. Information extraction, feature evaluation, and classification algorithms are, at this first level, used in the image preprocessing stage.

At the second level, the entity for information extraction and feature evaluation is the cell image as such. Cell image feature vectors are formed and classified.

At the third level, information pertaining to whole cell populations is analyzed. The data sets could be all cells collected from a given patient or all cells from a population given some treatment. Again, the cell population is characterized by certain features such as (a) the proportional composition of cells of different cell types, (b) proportion of cells showing certain degrees of response, (c) numbers of cells from different subpopulations, or (d) degrees of atypicality (Reinhardt et al., 1979). At this level of analysis, one is interested in assigning either a patient or a cell population to a given class such as a diagnostic entity or a type of response. Features for the cell population thus have to be computed and evaluated and a cell-population feature vector formed. These may then be classified or clustered.

The only problem-specific programs are the feature extraction modules. Features are defined, computed, and filed in feature files; then feature evaluation and selection, the forming of feature vectors, and feature-vector classification are accomplished by the same modules for each level of analysis. This process occurs whether the feature vectors represent image points, cell images, or cell populations.

A. Cell Image Features

The analysis of cell images may proceed through all of the following stages. First, during data acquisition, the cell image is recorded, digitized, and edited so that only the cell image itself in a clear background is stored in the computer. One may store the images in the form of arrays of transmission values or of optical densities. Data in the TICAS 11/45 system are stored as OD values because OD is directly and linearly proportional to the amounts of absorbing matter at each image point and the analysis is directed to an assessment of the spatial distribution patterns of DNA and other cytomorphometric properties relating to cell mass. All features are derived from the OD values. In converting transmission values to optical densities it is imperative that a sufficiently long reference table be used. Short tables of only 200 entries lead to wide gaps in the higher OD value sequence.

In the digitized images, the numerical values for the OD, typically measured on 0.5×0.5 μm^2 spots and at an appropriately selected wavelength, usually range in value from zero to 2.00 (Fig. 2). Since it is much

```
0   0   0   0   0   0   0   0   0   0   0   0   0   0   0   0   0   0   0   0   0
0   0   0   0   0   0   0   0   0   0   0   0   0   0   0   0   0   0   0   0   0
0   0   0   0   0   0   0   0   0   1   2   3   0   0   0   0   0   0   0   0   0
0   0   0   0   0   0   0   4  12  16  16  15   7   0   0   0   0   0   0   0   0
0   0   0   0   0   2  12  17  21  25  23  23  19  11  11   3   0   0   0   0   0
0   0   0   0   7  16  16  12  23  41  43  41  35  30  25  17   9   0   0   0   0
0   0   0   5  21  21  20  31  40  67  70  55  49  51  49  29  20   9   0   0   0
0   0   2  19  21  17  28  41  55  64  65  56  50  70  67  46  28  19   1   0   0
0   0   5  21  15  24  37  50  48  56  58  57  54  68  68  63  42  26  13   0   0
0   0  16  20  14  31  55  50  55  58  40  42  45  60  64  54  41  30  18   0   0
0   1  19  14  19  39  61  51  62  61  44  35  43  55  58  46  56  43  21   4   0
0   2  18  12  19  36  55  72  73  64  47  38  51  60  63  53  62  55  24   7   0
0   5  16  11  16  38  57  70  70  61  55  47  52  58  71  64  63  61  26  12   0
0   6  15  11  14  37  55  66  59  55  56  45  53  57  73  68  70  60  25  10   0
0   4  13  11   9  30  46  58  48  46  52  47  56  50  51  56  66  53  24   0   1
0   0  13  15  10  31  45  52  57  64  50  48  57  54  52  43  47  35  19   5   0
0   0   9  19  16  28  52  63  64  69  57  51  56  57  51  44  43  28  17   2   0
0   0   1  17  16  26  50  61  66  58  52  50  57  62  53  51  41  19  14   0   0
0   0   0   4  22  18  36  51  70  65  59  53  53  54  57  46  31  14   3   0   0
0   0   0   0  10  17  23  43  61  71  71  61  55  42  42  28  20   4   0   0   0
0   0   0   0   0   4  15  22  31  43  51  46  37  30  19   6   0   0   0   0   0
0   0   0   0   0   0   2   7  13  19  17  13  10   4   0   0   0   0   0   0   0
0   0   0   0   0   0   0   0   0   0   0   0   0   0   0   0   0   0   0   0   0
0   0   0   0   0   0   0   0   0   0   0   0   0   0   0   0   0   0   0   0   0
0   0   0   0   0   0   0   0   0   0   0   0   0   0   0   0   0   0   0   0   0
```

Total No. of Points = 286   Total OD   6646

FIGURE 2. Digitized image of a lymphocyte. Each value represents the optical density reading at a 0.5×0.5 μm^2 spot.

more economical to store integer numbers in a computer, it is customary to multiply all OD values by a factor of 100. The data-acquisition step may be followed by an image preprocessing step. Preprocessing may involve an image transformation and may have one or both of the following objectives: (a) An image transformation may make it easier to extract features. For example, a 3×3 point median smoothing algorithm is helpful for the finding of the nuclear boundary. (b) Image transformations using techniques such as erosions and dilatations may lead to transformed images of characteristic texture which exhibit accentuated differences and may provide finer diagnostic discrimination (Serra, 1974; Reinhardt *et al.*, 1979). Following preprocessing, the image itself, a transformed version thereof, or both are submitted to feature-extracting algorithms. The values for a predetermined feature set are stored on a disc file. From among the large number of computed features, those providing pertinent information have to be selected. Feature evaluation and selection eliminates a great many features from further consideration. The remaining features are now applied (a) to provide a set of numerically defined descriptive data for the cells, (b) to provide classification rules, (c) to test hypotheses according to given experimental designs, or (d) to examine the structure of the feature space in attempts to detect subsets of cells with significantly different chromatin distribution patterns.

The features which have been found useful for the analysis of chromatin distribution patterns fall into several groups.

1. There is a set of features which describe the cell image as a whole. They are therefore known as ''global features.'' Examples are the cell area, nuclear area, total OD of the cell, total OD of the nucleus, and the average OD of the nucleus.

2. The next set of features is derived from the first order statistics of the digitized values in a cell image. Examples are the relative frequencies of occurrence of OD values, i.e., the optical density histogram. The histogram may further be characterized by its descriptive statistics; such as the variance of OD values, the third, fourth, and higher moments about the mean OD value. The optical density histogram may be decomposed into distribution functions for values in the cytoplasm and values in the nucleus. Fig. 3 shows the OD histogram of Feulgen-stained human B cells, T cells, and monocytes (Durie *et al.*, 1978). The differences between B and T cells are less pronounced in Wright-stained preparations as seen in Fig. 4.

Figure 5 shows the histograms of OD values for human lymphocytes at times zero, 24, 48, and 72 h after stimulation with phytohemagglutinin (Bartels *et al.*, 1969a). It appears that a maximum response can be detected at 48 h and that the cells go through a cycle. The histogram for the transformed cells at 72 h closely resembles the initially observed histogram. The changes in histogram contour could be described by the moments about the

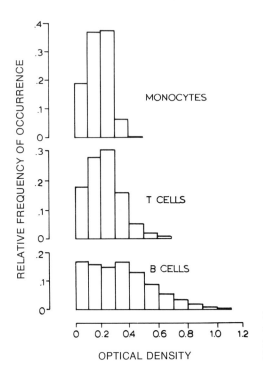

FIGURE 3. Distribution of optical density values from Feulgen-stained monocytes, T cells, and B cells from human subjects.

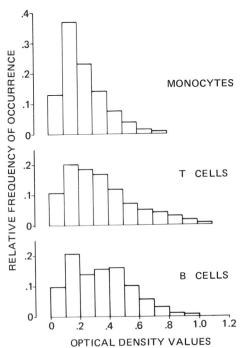

FIGURE 4. Distribution of optical density values from Wright-stained monocytes, T cells, and B cells from human subjects.

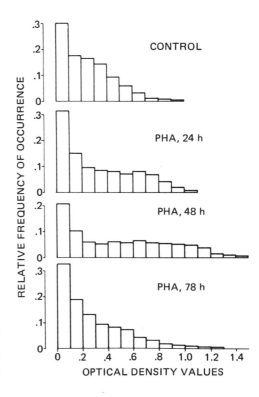

FIGURE 5. Distribution of optical density values for human lymphocytes after stimulation with phytohemagglutinin for various time periods. Cells were stained by the Feulgen procedure.

mean OD value (Table 1). The OD histogram may be fitted by a polynomial and the coefficients used to describe its contour. The OD histogram may similarly be described by a set of Fourier coefficients.

3. The transition probabilities for OD values between adjacent measuring points in the digitized cell image provide a set of image features which

TABLE 1

Evaluation of the Moments about the Mean OD value from Lymphocytes Stimulated *in Vitro* with Phytohemagglutinin

Time after stimulation (h)	Moments about the mean OD value		
	m_1	m_2	m_3
0	0.257	0.0412	0.0081
24	0.339	0.0836	0.0171
48	0.529	0.1723	0.0352
72	0.268	0.0574	0.0169

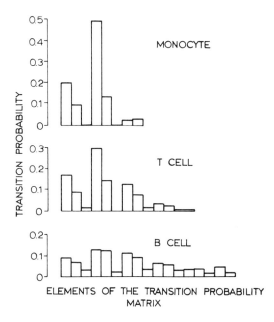

FIGURE 6. Distribution of the elements of the transition probability matrix from Feulgen-stained monocytes, T cells, and B cells from human subjects

involve second order statistics, i.e., for a Markovian dependence scheme involving only two immediately adjacent values (Bartels *et al.,* 1969b; Pressman, 1976a,b; Haralick *et al.,* 1973). It is usual to set up optical density ranges for the different states of the Markovian scheme so that they form equiprobable segments (Fig. 6). In this way, any information already offered by the first-order statistics in the OD histogram is eliminated.

One may use the transition probabilities themselves as features. One may also use descriptive statistics computed from the entire transition probability matrix, as suggested by Haralick (1973) and Pressman (1976a). Rosenfeld and Troy (1970) suggested computing the moment of inertia about the diagonal of a transition probability matrix. The coarser a texture is, the more likely neighboring image points are to fall into the same OD range. Values then will tend to congregate near the diagonal and the matrix will have a small moment of inertia.

4. Farther extending dependencies may be extracted from correlograms (Bartels *et al.,* 1974a). The correlation of values at a given point in the image to those of points one, two, three, or more points removed is computed (Fig. 7).

1. Run-Length Statistics

Run-length statistics have been adapted for texture analysis and have been used by a number of researchers (Bacus, 1970; Bradley, 1968; Landeweerd and Gelsema, 1978). A sequence of similar events is called a "run," for example, the sequence $+ + - + - - - + +$ is a sequence with five runs. In a random arrangement one would expect a large number of runs. There will be fewer runs when there is a systematic deviation from an assumed model. Run-length statistics lend themselves ideally to the definition of texture features. They have the potential for high discriminatory power. Run-length statistics are distribution-free. They can readily be implemented on a computer. They may be applied to the OD value sequence in the digitized image or to images converted to an array of differences. A typical application is as follows. For nuclei from a given population the median OD value is computed. Each image point then has the same *a priori* probability to fall into the OD range above or below the median. For a scan through any given cell from that population, one would expect a random sequence of values above and below the median. For cells from a different cell population, the median OD value may be quite different. Such scans would tend to produce sequences where many values above or below follow each other in a far-from-random fashion.

One may calculate the total number of runs, the length of the largest run, and other run-length statistics. The statistical test is one of randomness against sequential dependency. For given sample sizes, permutation theory provides exact probabilities for arrangements with at least one run of a given length, the number of runs of either kind, and, as a matter of fact, for each pattern of values above or below threshold. Either the run counts, or descriptive statistics thereof, or their probabilities of occurrence under the assumption of a certain model may be used as features.

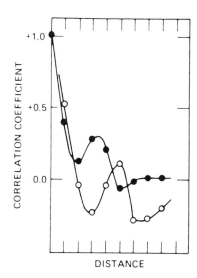

FIGURE 7. Correlogram for a sequence of optical density values centered in the nuclei of images from lymphocytes obtained from lymph nodes of patients with benign lymphadenitis (○) and from patients with malignant lymphoma (●).

2. Chromatin Condensation Indices

De Campos-Vidal *et al.* (1973) define three chromatin condensation indices. First, a criterion is chosen to set a threshold on the OD scale. All values below that threshold are considered as "noncondensed"; all values above are considered as "condensed" chromatin. The threshold criterion may be merely an arbitrarily chosen OD value. It may be chosen so that no more than a predetermined proportion of the nuclear area will fall into the noncondensed area, e.g., no more than 80%. In the latter instance the threshold is related to the histogram contour rather than to an absolute OD value.

The first index is defined as the average OD of the condensed chromatin divided by the average OD of all values of the nucleus. The second index assesses the peripheral tendency of the chromatin. It is defined as the averaged sum of the squared Euclidean distances of condensed chromatin points from the center of the cell. The third chromatin condensation index is a well-known measure from stereology (Fig. 8). It is the circumference of all condensed material divided by the area it occupies. This expression may be normalized. For a uniform chromatin distribution within a circle, a value of unity would be assumed.

3. Radial OD Profiles

The radial distribution of chromatin may be assessed by projection of all digitized OD values onto the radius. For this purpose, the digitized cell image is first converted to polar coordinates, a process which requires

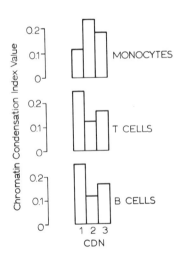

FIGURE 8.   Distribution of the three chromatin condensation indices from Feulgen-stained monocytes, T cells, and B cells from human subjects.

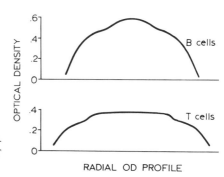

FIGURE 9. Distribution of the radial optical density profile from Feulgen-stained T cells and B cells from human subjects.

value interpolation. Then, at distances from the cell center corresponding to one, two, . . . , k measuring points, the optical density values are averaged. The result is a radial OD profile (Fig. 9).

4. Chromatin Texture

Chromatin texture may be assessed by an algorithm originally proposed by Vastola *et al.* (1974). It has been termed "waveform analysis." The basic algorithm is a "peak-finding" routine. The OD value sequence along a scan line is examined and converted to a difference line. For each point the OD value is compared to the preceding point. An increase in OD is marked as a +. If the value stays within the same OD range, it is marked as a 0. If the OD value decreases, it is marked as a −. A peak is defined either as the first point in a +− pair as seen in Fig. 10A or as the middle point of a sequence as shown in Fig. 10B. Segments of the difference line as shown above are called "waves." A wave starts with the nearest 0+ or −+ pair and ends with a +− or −0 for so-called "minimum waves." To detect large chromatin clumps, so-called "maximum waves" are defined; an example is given in Fig. 10C. The maximum wave starts with the 0 + sequence, and it may encompass a minimum wave for the last six points. Features derived from this wave algorithm are the number of points in a wave and the wave height which is found by connecting the start and end point and projecting the peak onto the baseline as shown in Fig. 10D. Next there is a set of features which describes the linking of waves between consecutive scan lines. Waves are considered "linked" if the peaks fall into the same column of the digitized image, or into the column immediately preceding or following the column with the first peak. Such a set of linked waves is called a "chain." If n is the number of links, $n-1$ is used as a feature. If the chain branches, the number from the longest branch is used. This is shown in Fig. 10D. Another feature is the chain width. For all waves

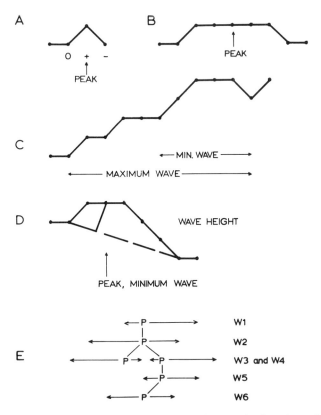

FIGURE 10. Peak finding and chaining of waves. (A) Characterization of a peak. (B) Characterization of a peak. (C) Characterization of minimum and maximum waves. (D) Characterization of the height of a wave. (E) Chaining of waves. Only waves whose peaks occur in register or in columns immediately adjacent are considered as chained. Branching is allowed.

linked by a chain the number of points are averaged. An analogous feature is derived from the wave heights and is referred to as the chain height. Other features are derived from the frequency of occurrence of chains of length 2,3,4, . . . , etc. Finally, there are features derived from the average ratio of chain width to chain length, height to width, and fraction of total nuclear area occupied by chains of a certain minimum length.

5. OD Meshwork Analysis

Extensions of the wave and chain analyses into the OD range have become known as meshwork analysis. The wave analysis as outlined above may be carried out for a number of OD intervals; the histograms of the feature values as a function of the OD range are then calculated.

6. The Texture Tree

The forming of a "texture tree" is the first step in a texture analysis program as suggested by Simon *et al.* (1975). For different OD ranges, the number of immediately adjacent image points falling into the same OD range are recorded and arranged in a hierarchic order to form a tree graph. The ordinate represents the OD scale. The tree is then, in a further data-reduction step, plotted as a texture curve, where the number of "nodes" are plotted over the OD scale. The OD levels for which the nodes are established do not have to follow a linear scale. Features derived from the texture tree are the root length, i.e., the OD level where the first branching occurs; another feature is the OD level range from the first branch to the OD level of the densest image point. The number of "leaves" on the tree, i.e., of areas of distinct OD levels, is used as a feature as is the average OD of the entire tree after the first branching threshold is subtracted. The distribution of average OD level in each leaf is defined as a set of features and the ratio of the geometric average to the arithmetic average of area differences at each OD level. Finally, the proportions of the total area at each OD level are used as features and the number of relative maxima on the texture curve. Table 2 shows the data for which the texture curve in Fig. 11 is plotted.

7. Granulometric Analysis

Granulometric analysis relies on a number of features which are directly derived from the chromatin granules. These features include (a) the number of granules, (b) the area occupied by them, (c) their size distribution, and (d) their compactness as determined by circumference to area

TABLE 2
Data for Texture Tree Analysis

OD level	Number of branches	Accumulated area	Difference
0.00	1	100	17
0.40	1	83	53
0.60	2	30	19
0.80	3	11	10
1.00	1	1	1

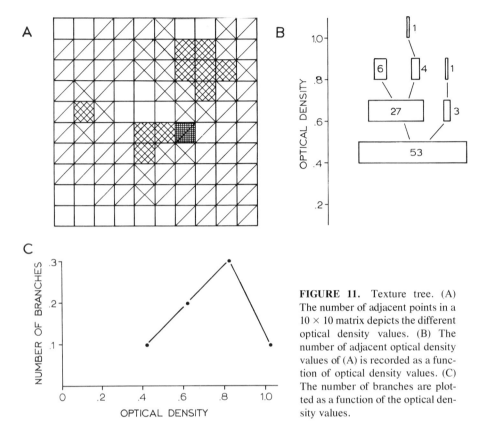

FIGURE 11. Texture tree. (A) The number of adjacent points in a 10 × 10 matrix depicts the different optical density values. (B) The number of adjacent optical density values of (A) is recorded as a function of optical density values. (C) The number of branches are plotted as a function of the optical density values.

measurements (Fig. 12). These algorithms trace around a granule as defined by the OD threshold. The better algorithms have the capacity of backtracking to exclude "holes" or empty areas from the granule size determination. Granulometric analysis often requires 0.25μm step size resolution.

Another approach to granule tracing was published by Wasmund (1976). It is designed to acquire the data as each scan line is recorded. The algorithm labels each new intercepted particle with an index number. When, in a new scan line, an intercept is found to be directly registered with an index number in the preceding scan line, that intercept is given the same index number. When two different index numbers are assigned on the same scan line to two immediately adjacent locations, the entire field with the higher index number is reindexed to the lower index number. In this fashion, particles or granules with concave shapes are identified as one and the same granule. The process is shown in Fig. 13. Granulometric features rest directly on higher order textural properties of the digitized image. A "granule" implies the occurrence of a whole group of points which are directly adjacent to each other and all in the same OD range. Features of this kind lend themselves ideally to the definition of secondary features which can be tailor-made to have high discrimination for a given pair of cell categories. The process may be called an induction of higher-order texture and it is best described by the following example. One may examine the OD histograms from two cell populations and compare their contours. An OD threshold is chosen so that, for example, for one cell population the top 25% of all points is retained and a much smaller proportion of points in the other cell population is retained. For the histogram features, i.e., the first-order statistics above the threshold, the discrimination is not affected. Also, the threshold may have only a minimal effect on the number and size of granules in the first cell population. However, in the second cell population, occurrence of a value above the threshold is now a rare event, following Poisson statistics. The setting of the threshold has a dramatic effect on the remaining number of granules, and especially on their size distribution. The higher-order statistical properties of the second cell population are thus selectively changed to maximize the difference between it and the first cell population.

The introduction of such topographic effects has also been the basis for the equiprobability contour procedure used to discriminate between cell populations (Bartels *et al.*, 1968). Here, the OD histogram from one cell population is used to define a certain band of OD values. These can be expected to appear in a certain topographic pattern in cell images of that

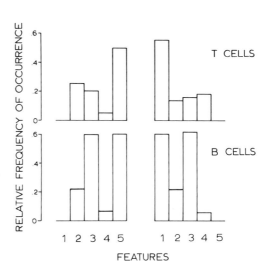

FIGURE 12. Granularity assessment for Feulgen-stained B and T cells from human subjects. The first set of five features expresses the relative frequencies of occurrence of granules in five size classes. The second set of five features represents the relative frequencies of occurrence of granules with different ratios of granule area to granule perimeter length.

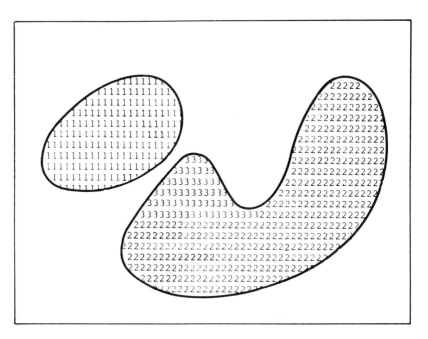

FIGURE 13. Granulometric analysis. Depicted is the operation of a tagging algorithm in which the next step would be to rename all "3" points in the granule as "2" points.

class. In cell images from a different cell category, and with a different OD histogram contour, the superposition of that same OD band will lead to distinctively different topographic point patterns (Fig. 14). One may perform such an equiprobability contour mapping as a preprocessing operation resulting in a specifically transformed image. From these images one can extract feature values such as radial profile data.

Changes in the higher order statistics of the digitized cell image are also introduced by linear filtering techniques.* Linear filters may be defined and optimized to enhance the granularity in a given spatial frequency range, e.g., in the 0.5-μm or the 2-μm granule size range. A linear filtering operation, done as a preprocessing step will yield a transformed image. For cells of a type where 0.5-μm granules predominate such filtering will lead to a transformed image with markedly different texture from what will be found when the same filter is applied to a cell type characterized by 2-μm granules.

*Abmayer, W., Burger, G. and Soost, H. J. Progress Report for the TUDAB Project for Automated Cancer cell detection. Paper presented at the Sixth Engineering Foundation Conference on Automated Cytology, April 23–29, 1978, Schloss Elmau, Federal Republic of Germany, and accepted for publication in the *Journal of Histochemistry and Cytochemistry*.

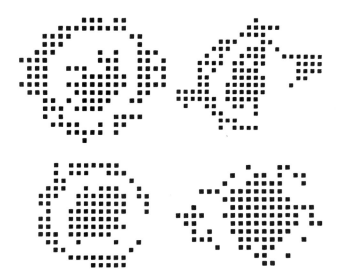

Figure 14. Equiprobability map for cells from human epidermoid carcinoma. Two optical density ranges are shown; (a) 0.01 to 0.16 OD and (b) 0.70 to 1.60 OD. The topographic distribution is characterized by a core of points of 0.70–1.60 OD values, surrounded by a ring of values from the lower OD range.

The effects of a linear filtering are best illustrated by an example. The demonstrated filter forms the second derivative of the original digitized image; it is a Laplace transform filter. For demonstration purposes, only a one-dimensional filter will be given as an example. The filter shall be specified as follows: −1 +2 −1. Let it be assumed that the following value sequence in the original image is to be processed:

$$11 \quad 10 \quad 12 \quad 22 \quad 10 \quad 8 \quad 6$$

Note the "granule" at the high value of 22. Moving the filter over this value sequence leads to the following transformation:

11	10	12	transforms to	−11	20	−12	averaged =	−3
10	12	22		−10	24	−22		−8
12	22	10		−12	44	−10		+22
22	10	8		−22	20	−8		−10
10	8	6		−10	16	−12		−6

To avoid negative entries, it is customary to add a constant to every value. In this example addition of a value of 20 to the averaged transformed image gives an image transformation of:

$$17 \quad 12 \quad 42 \quad 10 \quad 14$$

The new values no longer represent optical densities as such. One can see that the transformed value sequence emphasizes the "granule."

8. Spectral Data and Features

Spectral information has in the past been used primarily for the purposes of scene segmentation and delineation of nuclear and cytoplasmic boundaries (Taylor *et al.*, 1978b). One might consider these uses as image preprocessing. Typical features for image point vectors would be derived from combinations of spatial and spectral gradients, e.g., the difference in OD at a given wavelength between two adjacent image points relative to the difference in OD between the same two image points at another wavelength. However, work in clinical cytology has shown that spectral features computed for either the nuclear region or the cytoplasm offer valuable diagnostic clues (Reale *et al.*, 1979). Of particular interest here are spectral contrasts, such as the difference between the OD in the red and in the green spectral region divided by the sum of these two ODs (Taylor *et al.*, 1978b). By comparing contrasts of this kind only for certain bands in the equiprobable divided OD histogram, some aspects of spectral texture are brought out. An example is a feature such as the median OD in the 75%–100% cumulative-frequency-distribution (cfd) range of the red spectral region, minus the median OD in the 25%- to 50%-cfd range of the blue spectral region, divided by the standard deviation of OD values in the red region, 75%–100% cfd. It is clear that the possibilities for combining descriptive measures into features are numerous. Some rationale for defining a given feature should prevail. All of the textural feature sets described above may be extended into the spectral domain: the OD histograms, the Markovian dependence schemes, the correlograms, the condensation indices, the granularity measures, and the run-statistics features. In particular, features derived from run statistics lend themselves to the simultaneous consideration of OD values in the same or in different image points at different wavelengths. However, transitions between OD ranges in different spectral ranges may just as readily be defined for spectral Markov features.

9. Shape Features

Shape features offer the advantage that as a rule they are not greatly affected by slight differences in staining (Young *et al.*, 1974; Sychra *et al.*, 1976, 1977). In the study of lymphocyte populations, shape features have not been used to a significant degree. Shape features which may be applicable and which have been successfully employed in the analysis of cellular materials are (a) features assessing the roundness of the nucleus, (b) features assessing the presence and extent of indentations, (c) features based on the ellipticity and convexity of the nucleus, and (d) features which provide a general description of shape, such as a set of Fourier coefficients. There are also measures of the regularity of the nuclear boundary, e.g., the variance of the difference chain code.

This latter feature is best illustrated by an example. A chain code is essentially a list of directions. When used to encode a nuclear boundary, each code element specifies the direction in which one has to proceed by one measuring spot distance to find the next boundary point. Figure 15 shows a set of directions and the associated code elements. A difference chain code is formed merely by taking the difference between two code elements. When an outline is convex and smooth, all elements of its difference chain code tend to be the same or at least close. The variance of these elements thus would be small. An irregular outline will lead to abrupt and large directional changes and thus to large values in the difference chain code and a high variance of these numbers.

10. Probabilistically Defined Features

As an example for a probabilistically defined feature, the "tolerance level" for an optical density histogram shall be demonstrated. The operator first defines an OD histogram. This may be taken from a given cell popula-

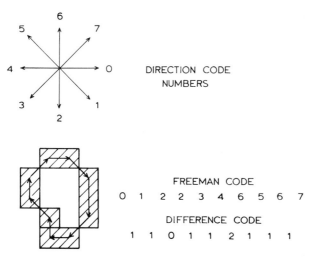

FIGURE 15.   Chain codes may be employed to define shape features for a nuclear boundary.

TABLE 3
Printout of Results from Tolerance Regions Program for Virus-Altered Murine Lymphocytes

```
INPUT OPTIONS:

1...READ IN POPULATION HISTOGRAM FROM FEATURE FILE
2...MANUAL INPUT OF INDIVIDUAL HISTOGRAM
3...READ IN FREQUENCY HISTOGRAM FILE

OPTION NUMBER:   3
ACCEPT?  Y
ENTER NAME OF HISTOGRAM FILE IN A6<AAAAAA>:   M134FS
ACCEPT?  Y

DO YOU WANT TO SAVE THE RESULTS?  N
ACCEPT?  Y


PROTOTYPE 1SPRO1
TOLERANCE REGION = 95.00
```

CELL ID	POSITION INSIDE	POSITION OUTSIDE	CALCULATED TOLERANCE LEVEL
1	IN		44.60
2		OUT	99.52
3	IN		22.56
4	IN		20.43
5	IN		8.64
6	IN		1.00
7	IN		1.00
8	IN		92.17
9	IN		75.73
10		OUT	99.52
11	IN		1.00

tion or the operator may enter the relative frequencies of occurrence for every interval manually. This histogram is called the prototype. One then may read in a file of histogram data and test whether each histogram falls into a set tolerance region for the prototype, i.e., 95%-tolerance region. The calculated tolerance level for each histogram may be used as a histogram feature. It is a distance measure and expresses what proportion of cells is closer to the prototype than the cell in question. For example, in Table 3, cell ID 2 has a tolerance level of 99.52. This means that only 0.48%, or roughly one cell in 200 has a histogram as different from the prototype as this cell. The smaller the number which is calculated for the tolerance level, the more typical a representative of the prototype is the cell in question.

B. Statistical Evaluation of the Data

Statistical analysis of the data in cell image analysis enters at several levels. For certain cell image features which can be visually observed by cytologists, one may wish to determine the mean values, their variance and possible changes due to treatment. When the differences are small and not obvious after mere inspection, one may wish to secure any experimentally determined differences by an analysis of variance. Proper experimental design in analysis of variance can lead to substantial economy in data collection. However, we have not found it useful to have extensive analysis of variance programs on the computer because two experimental situations are rarely alike. Rather, for each data set the basic data needed in any experimental design can be printed out. These can readily be arranged into the most effective design for: a factorial arrangement of treatments, nested designs, or a simple one-way or two-way anova design. A sample printout of this program is shown in Table 4. The data represent the values for three scaled chromatin condensation indices for a set of mouse B lymphocytes. Data may be presented in visual form by selecting two features for the data sets and analyzing them as bivariate distributions. One may compute the bivariate mean vector, the confidence ellipse for the bivariate mean and the tolerance region. Since the practical application usually involves demonstrating some difference between different data sets and one is interested in one's ability to assign a cell to one or another category, the program computes the Bayesian boundary. This marks the line on which assignment of a two-dimensional cell feature vector to either category would be equally likely. The Bayesian boundary is placed so that the risk of an erroneous assignment is equalized for the two categories. Table 5 shows a sample program run. The two chosen cell categories are mouse T and B lymphocytes and the two chosen features are nuclear area and the value of a discriminant function. The program first provides some descriptive statistics for the bivariate distributions as shown for the T cells. A similar set of statistics is calculated for the B cells. Two display options exist. One display presents each cell's bivariate vector and the Bayesian boundary (Fig.

TABLE 4
Sample Printout of Information for Use in Analysis of Variance Programs

FILE NAME: M2B100. CNS
TOTAL CELLS: 126

FEATURE NAME	MEAN	SUM OF X	SUM OF X^2	$\dfrac{<SUMX>^2}{N}$	STAND. DEV.
CNS1-1	0.1362E 00	0.1717E 02	0.234703E 01	0.233855E 01	0.823467E-02
CNS2	0.1742E 00	0.2194E 02	0.385020E 01	0.382188E 01	0.150531E-01
CNS3-2	0.1394E 00	0.1756E 02	0.245261E 01	0.244792E 01	0.612852E-02

TABLE 5
Printout of Results for Bivariate Plot for Two Feature Files of Mouse T and B Cells

```
FILE NAMES ARE:
M2T100
M2B100

FEATURES USED:
ARE-2
SDMF1

A PRIORI PROBABILITY FOR CELLS TO FALL INTO FILE M2T100 IS:  0.50

A PRIORI PROBABILITY FOR CELLS TO FALL INTO FILE M2B100 IS:  0.50

DISPLAY CHARACTER OF FILE M2T100 = T

DISPLAY CHARACTER OF FILE M2B100 = B

FOR FILE M2T100:

# OF CELLS:  126
SAMPLE MEAN:                1.2934              0.9280
STANDARD DEV.:              0.1755              0.3636
COVARIANCE:     0.3528E-01
CORRELATION COEFF.:  0.5528

EIGENVALUES:   0.1433E 00   0.1975E-01

SLOPE OF PRINCIPAL AXIS:      0.3137
        MINOR AXIS:          -3.1873
95% CONFIDENCE LIMITS OF MAJOR SLOPE:        0.233        0.399

COORDINATES FOR 95% CONFIDENCE ELLIPSE OF BIVARIATE MEAN
              X VALUE                  Y VALUE
              1.3260                   0.9280
              1.2609                   0.9280
              1.2934                   0.9955
              1.2934                   0.8606
              1.3186                   1.0084
              1.2682                   0.8477
              1.2636                   0.9374
              1.3233                   0.9187

PROBABILITY DENSITY OF TOLERANCE REGION ELLIPSE =  0.5000
              X VALUE                  Y VALUE
              1.4738                   0.9280
              1.1130                   0.9280
              1.2934                   1.3016
              1.2934                   0.5544
              1.4331                   1.3734
              1.1537                   0.4827
              1.1281                   0.9799
              1.4587                   0.8762
```

16). The second display shows the bivariate population mean, confidence ellipses, tolerance ellipses, and the Bayesian boundary (Fig. 17).

C. Feature Evaluation and Selection

The preceding section describes a substantial number of features, all of which express some aspect of chromatin distribution. For a given cell analysis problem a small subset of these features is usually quite sufficient.

Feature-evaluation algorithms may be used to determine which features are most valuable for a given task. In the TICAS 11/45 program package, feature evaluation is carried out in stages.

1. Kruskal–Wallis Test

In a first stage, a fast and nonparametric statistical test, the Kruskal–Wallis test, is employed to screen the feature files for features that show statistically significant differences between two data sets (Bradley, 1968). The Kruskal–Wallis test algorithm first merges the feature values from two cell data sets. The values are then ranked and each feature value is replaced by its rank order number. If the feature values from one of the data sets are consistently higher or lower than those from the other data set, their aver-

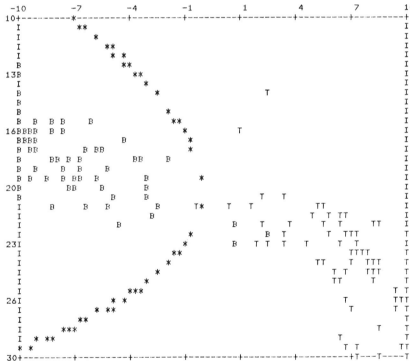

FIGURE 16. Computer printout of a bivariate mean plot for two features for Feulgen-stained murine T and B cells. Symbols T and B represent the cells. Asterisks represent Bayesian decision boundary.

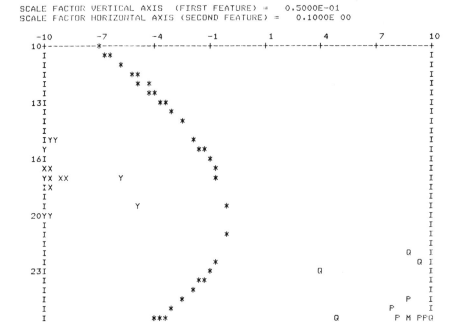

SCALE FACTOR VERTICAL AXIS (FIRST FEATURE) = 0.5000E-01
SCALE FACTOR HORIZONTAL AXIS (SECOND FEATURE) = 0.1000E 00

FIGURE 17. Computer printout of the bivariate plot shown in Fig. 16. Asterisks represent Bayesian decision boundary. M represents bivariate means for the T cells; P and X represent the confidence ellipses for the T and B cells; and Q and Y represent the tolerance ellipses for T- and B-cell populations.

aged rank order numbers will reflect this difference. The test is distribution-free, i.e., no assumptions are made with respect to the distribution of feature values in either data set. The algorithm is very fast. It returns the value of a test statistic H, and a value for the level of significance of any difference between data sets. As a rule, the Kruskal–Wallis test allows one to dismiss 80% of all computed features and to identify typically about 20 to 50 features as worthy of further consideration. Table 6 shows the results of a Kruskal–Wallis test for 18 OD histogram features, for cell area and total OD, and three chromatin condensation indices. The discrimination task was the recognition of Feulgen-stained human B cells from monocytes. Values of all alpha (cumulative probability) smaller than 0.05 indicate that statistically significant differences exist between the feature values of the

TABLE 6
Printout of Results of Kruskal–Wallis Test for 23 Features for the Discrimination of Human
B Cells and Monocytes

KRUSKAL-WALLIS TEST PERFORMED ON B CELLS AND MONOCYTES:

FEATURE	FEATURE NO	TEST STATISTICS H	CUMULATIVE PROBABILITY
BIN1[1]	1	16.35	0.000--0.005
BIN2	2	138.4	0.000--0.005
BIN3	3	120.1	0.000--0.005
BIN4	4	2.657	0.100--0.250
BIN5	5	89.79	0.000--0.005
BIN6	6	147.7	0.000--0.005
BIN7	7	128.6	0.000--0.005
BIN8	8	79.65	0.000--0.005
BIN9	9	54.70	0.000--0.005
BIN10	10	39.23	0.000--0.005
BIN11	11	32.48	0.000--0.005
BIN12	12	15.87	0.000--0.005
BIN13	13	7.170	0.005--0.010
BIN14	14	0.9999	0.250--0.500
BIN15	15	0.9999	0.250--0.500
BIN16	16	0.0000	0.900--1.000
BIN17	17	0.0000	0.900--1.000
BIN18	18	0.0000	0.900--1.000
AREA	19	166.1	0.000--0.005
TE	20	31.59	0.000--0.005
AVG OD	21	180.4	0.000--0.005
CND1	22	5.612	0.010--0.025
CND2	23	160.3	0.000--0.005

[1]BIN and HIST are equivalent terms.

two compared distributions. The average OD, the nuclear area, and the chromatin condensation index CND2 render the highest values for the test statistic H; a plot of two of these features reveals that they alone would provide for good discrimination (Fig. 18).

2. Receiver Operating Characteristic Curve

Statistical differences between two feature value distributions are a necessary but not a sufficient condition: it does not guarantee good discrimination.

The second stage of the feature evaluation program, therefore, examines the feature's ability to discriminate. Discrimination capability of a single feature is measured by the "measure of detectability" d' from the

```
                           SCATTER DIAGRAM
                           AVG   VS  CND2

          0.1663                0.3106                0.4549
          !**********!**********!**********!**********!**********!    B   M
  15.36   *                      M                               *   0   1
  16.34   *                M                           M     M  *   0   3
  17.31   *               M     M                    M          *   0   3
  18.29   *        M   MM M   M        MM    M     MM            *   0  11
  19.27   *      M MMM  MMM  MMM  M  M      M  M                 *   0  19
  20.24   *            MM    MM MM M         M                   *   0  13
  21.22   *      M M   MM   M M M M M           M               *   0  14
  22.19   *       M MM M  MMMMMM                                *   0  14
  23.17   *         M   MM MM     M                    M         *   0   8
  24.15   *         M MM            M M     M                    *   0   8
  25.12   * B       MMMM              M     M                    *   1   8
  26.10   *    MM     M     M    M M    M                        *   0   7
  27.07   *B         M      M     M                              *   1   3
  28.05   *        MMM     MM                                    *   0   5
  29.02   * BBB         MBM   M                                  *   5   4
  30.00   * B  B  B  B      M  M                                 *   5   2
  30.98   * B  B  BBBB                                           *   9   0
  31.95   *     BBBB   M    M                                    *   5   2
  32.93   *BBBB  BB                                              *   8   0
  33.90   *BB  BBB    BB                                         *  12   0
  34.88   *BBBB  B      B                                        *  10   0
  35.86   *BB  BMB                                               *   6   1
  36.83   *BBBB   B   B                                          *  11   0
  37.81   *B  BB     B                                           *   5   0
  38.78   *  BBBB           B                                    *   6   0
  39.76   *BBB  B  B                                             *   7   0
  40.74   *BB     B  B                                           *   5   0
  41.71   *BBBB                                                  *   8   0
  42.69   *  B  B  B      B                                      *   5   0
  43.66   *  BB   B  BB                                          *   5   0
  44.64   *B       B                                             *   2   0
  45.62   *  BB                                                  *   2   0
  46.59   *   B  B                                               *   3   0
  47.57   *  BB                                                  *   3   0
  48.54   *                                                      *   0   0
  49.52   *                                                      *   0   0
  50.50   * B                                                    *   1   0
  51.47   *                                                      *   0   0
  52.45   *                                                      *   0   0
  53.42   * B                                                    *   1   0
          !**********!**********!**********!**********!**********!
```

FIGURE 18. Computer printout of a scatter diagram showing the distribution of Feulgen-stained monocytes and B cells of human subjects, features selected by the Kruskal–Wallis test.

receiver operating characteristic curve (Sherwood *et al.*, 1976). It is derived as follows. If, between two feature value distributions, a decision threshold were set up, two types of error may occur. An observation from the first distribution may fall above the threshold and be classified as belonging to data set II. *Vice versa*, the distribution of values from data set II will extend to values below the threshold, and an item from distribution II may be classified as belonging to data set I. The magnitude of both errors depends directly on where one sets the threshold. If we denote the probability of finding a value above threshold for an item from distribution I as alpha, and the probability of finding for the same threshold setting an item from distribution II to have a value smaller than the threshold value as beta, then 1 − beta is the probability of correctly classifying an object from distribution II.

A plot of 1 − beta over alpha is known as the ROC curve (receiver operating characteristic curve). The area between this curve and the diagonal of the plot is known as the "measure of detectability" d'. If the curve coincides with the diagonal, the two distributions overlap completely and are identical. There is no discrimination and d' is equal to zero. Under ideal discrimination, alpha is zero and 1 − beta reaches a value of unity. The ROC curve reaches all the way into the upper left–most corner of the diagram and the full area of the upper triangle lies under the curve: d', then, assumes its highest possible value of 0.5, indicating complete discrimination. This measure of detectability can only be computed for a single feature at a time. An example is shown in Fig. 19. This is a classification problem involving Feulgen-stained B cells, T cells, and monocytes. The first decision node calls for a separation into either B cells or T cells plus monocytes. The figure shows the evaluation of the feature "nuclear area" for this discrimination task. The d' value of 0.319 indicates that this feature offers good discrimination potential. Features with a d' of less than 0.2 are generally not sufficiently effective. Table 7 shows the d' values for OD histogram data for the discrimination of Feulgen-stained human B cells from monocytes.

3. Ambiguity function

The discrimination potential of several features taken in combination may be assessed by the use of an ambiguity function (Genchi and Mori, 1965). The ambiguity function by Genchi and Mori (1965) is essentially an information measure. The function assumes a value of unity when no discrimination is possible, and a value of zero when error-free classification can be expected. It is computed as

$$A = - \sum^{c_j} \sum^{y_i} \Pr(c_j) \Pr(y_i|c_j) \log_N \Pr(y_i|c_j)$$

where A is the ambiguity, $\Pr(c_j)$ is the probability for the occurrence of a value in interval j; $\Pr(y_i|c_j)$ is the probability to be a member of category i given a feature value j has been observed. N is the number of cell categories. Results of a sample run for the human B cell and monocyte data are shown in Table 8. The ambiguity values for each of the relative frequencies of occurrence of OD, taken singly, are computed. For each, the range of values was divided into six intervals. This provided good estimates of the ambiguity. When more features are taken as a group, core restrictions may force one to restrict the number of intervals to a lesser number.

TABLE 7
Printout of Results of ROC Analysis for 18 Histogram Features for the Discrimination of Human B Cells and Monocytes

```
            ROC-CURVE d' VALUE FOR FILES:
            BCELL .HST AND MONO .HST
```

FEATURE NAME	ROC d'
BIN1 [1]	0.1664
BIN2	0.4077
BIN3	0.3030
BIN4	0.0233
BIN5	0.2894
BIN6	0.3245
BIN7	0.2578
BIN8	0.1783
BIN9	0.1314
BIN10	0.0999
BIN11	0.0994
BIN12	0.0798
BIN13	0.0440
BIN14	0.0025
BIN15	0.0000
BIN16	0.0000
BIN17	0.0000
BIN18	0.0000

[1]BIN and HIST are equivalent terms.

The calculation of an ambiguity value proceeds through the following steps. The range of values for the feature in both data sets is divided into a number of intervals. The number of observations falling into each interval (j) from data set K and from data set L and the combined total for each interval are listed below.

Interval j	dn group K	dn group L	Total
1	135	50	185
2	392	154	546
3	221	406	627
4	153	342	495
5	99	48	147
	1000	1000	2000

Next, the probabilities of occurrence are computed. The first column

ROC CURVE FOR ARN
PERFORMED ON TMDRW1 AND BDRW1

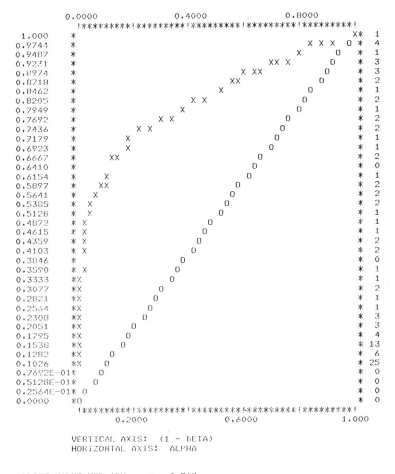

FIGURE 19.   Computer printout of a ROC curve of Feulgen-stained T and B cells from
human subjects analyzed for differences in relative nuclear area.

below [Pr(j)] lists the relative frequency of occurrence of events in each
interval j as computed from the column of totals listed above. Then, the
probability that an observation came from data set K, given it fell into
interval j is computed and the same is done for data set L. For example,
$Pr(K|1) = 135/185 = 0.7297$.

		$i = K$	$i = L$
j	$Pr\{j\}$	$Pr(K\vert j)$	$Pr(L\vert j)$
1	0.0925	0.7297	0.2703
2	0.2730	0.7179	0.2820
3	0.3135	0.3524	0.6475
4	0.2475	0.3090	0.6909
5	0.0735	0.6734	0.3265

We now need the value of $\log_N Pr(i\vert j)$, since we have two groups, $N = 2$.

TABLE 8
Printout of Results from Ambiguity Function Program Using Histogram Data Files of Human B Cells and Monocytes

```
INPUT FILE # 1     NAME:  BCELL     DATA POINTS:  126
INPUT FILE # 2     NAME:  MONO      DATA POINTS:  126

TOTAL # OF FEATURES:  18
TOTAL # OF DATA POINTS:  252

        2 GROUPS TO BE DISTINGUISHED
    GROUP  1 HAS  126 DATA POINTS
    GROUP  2 HAS  126 DATA POINTS
    # OF FEATURE VALUE INTERVAL =    6
    METHOD OF FORMING INTERVALS =    1

WEIGHT FACTOR FOR EACH GROUP:
GROUP #      FACTOR
    1         1.00
    2         1.00
```

FEATURE NAME	AMBIGUITY VALUE
BIN1	0.8997
BIN2	0.4880
BIN3	0.5743
BIN4	0.9049
BIN5	0.6798
BIN6	0.5058
BIN7	0.6096
BIN8	0.7430
BIN9	0.8247
BIN10	0.8693
BIN11	0.9112
BIN12	0.9507
BIN13	0.9758
BIN14	0.9960
BIN15	0.9960
BIN16	1.0000
BIN17	1.0000
BIN18	1.0000

These values are found by looking up $\log_{10} \Pr(i|j)$ and dividing it by $\log_{10} 2$. The calculations are

		$\Pr(i|j)$	$\log_{10} \Pr(i|j)$	$\log_2 \Pr(i|j)$
$i = K$		0.7297	-0.1370	-0.4551
		0.7179	-0.1441	-0.4787
		0.3524	-0.4530	-1.5049
		0.3090	-0.5101	-1.6946
		0.6734	-0.1718	-0.5707
$i = L$		0.2703	-0.5682	-1.8877
		0.2820	-0.5498	-1.8265
		0.6475	-0.1888	-0.6272
		0.6909	-0.1606	-0.5335
		0.3265	-0.4861	-1.6149

Logarithms have to be taken of numbers smaller than 1.00; an example may be helpful:

$$\log_{10} 0.7297 = (\log 7.297) - 1$$
$$= 0.8630 - 1$$
$$= -0.1370$$

We are now ready to compute the terms and form the double sum.

$j = 1$	$i = K$	$0.0925 \times 0.7297 \times -0.4551$	$=$	-0.03071
	$i = L$	$0.0925 \times 0.2703 \times -1.8877$	$=$	-0.04719
$j = 2$	$i = K$	$0.2730 \times 0.7179 \times -0.4787$	$=$	-0.0938
	$i = L$	$0.2730 \times 0.2820 \times -1.8265$	$=$	-0.1406
$j = 3$	$i = K$	$0.3135 \times 0.3524 \times -1.5049$	$=$	-0.06625
	$i = L$	$0.3135 \times 0.6475 \times -0.6272$	$=$	-0.12731
$j = 4$	$i = K$	$0.2475 \times 0.3090 \times -1.6946$	$=$	-0.12959
	$i = L$	$0.2475 \times 0.6909 \times -0.5335$	$=$	-0.09122
$j = 5$	$i = K$	$0.0735 \times 0.6734 \times -0.5707$	$=$	-0.02824
	$i = L$	$0.0735 \times 0.3265 \times -1.6149$	$=$	-0.03875
			$A =$	0.89366

The ambiguity A is 0.89366. A high value of d' and a low value for the ambiguity alone will not guarantee that one will obtain an effective selection of features. One wants to avoid features which have high correlation.

4. FMERIT *Function*

Addition of a feature which is highly correlated to the features already selected adds little new information, and thus may not improve the discrimination. In the TICAS 11/45 program package, a merit function is computed to circumvent this difficulty. The value is computed in two stages. First the values of d' and of A are combined into an intermediate value by the expression $[(1-A) + 2d']/2$.

The feature with the highest intermediate value is selected. The next feature is chosen from among those with high intermediate values so that the averaged correlation between the new feature and the already selected feature set is kept at a minimum. The merit function value follows from:

$$\frac{(1 - A) + 2d' + (1 - \bar{r})}{3}$$

For example, a feature with a high A, say $A = 0.95$, and a low measure of detectability, say $d' = 0.12$ would render a low intermediate value $[(1 - 0.95) + 0.24]/2 = 0.145$; if it would also lead to a high averaged correlation with the other already selected variables, say $\bar{r} = 0.80$, a low merit function value would result:

$$\frac{(1 - 0.95) + 2 \times 0.12 + (1 - 0.80)}{3} = 0.163$$

A sample run presenting the first few lines of a printout for the discrimination of mouse T and B lymphocytes is shown in Table 9.

D. Supervised Learning Algorithms

The selected features are then submitted to the various supervised learning algorithms. These algorithms may (a) make a further selection of a subset of features, (b) assign weights, (c) optimize the weights to obtain an overall minimized number of classification errors, and (d) set thresholds and establish an order in which the features are considered. In every case the supervised learning algorithms and the classification algorithms will derive and test a classification rule. This rule is stored on a disc under a suitably chosen file name. Three examples of supervised learning algorithms are described.

1. Algorithm DSELECT

The first is the algorithm DSELECT, of the original TICAS program package (Bartels and Bellamy, 1970; Bartels et al., 1970). The algorithm requires two feature files, one for each "training set" of cell images. The algorithm is restricted to two category discrimination problems. It proceeds

TABLE 9

Partial Listing of Results from FMERIT Function Test of Murine T and B Lymphocytes

```
FILE NAMES ARE:   M2T100 and M2B100
NUMBER OF TOTAL FEATURES USED = 74
NUMBER OF BEST FEATURES WANTED = 15
```

FEATURE NAME	AMBIGUITY VALUE	ROC VALUE	INTERMEDIATE VALUE
1. BIN1	0.89075	0.20383	0.25846
2. BIN2	0.70822	0.34266	0.48855
3. BIN3	0.63964	0.36798	0.54816
4. BIN4	0.82383	0.24915	0.33723
5. BIN5	0.88115	0.01846	0.07788
6. BIN6	0.62138	0.26997	0.45928
7. BIN7	0.53639	0.30212	0.53393
8. BIN8	0.65866	0.28345	0.45412
9. BIN9	0.77486	0.19177	0.30434
10. BIN10	0.85501	0.08422	0.15671
11. BIN11	0.96845	-0.02740	-0.01163
12. BIN12	1.00000	0.00000	0.00000
13. BIN13	1.00000	0.00000	0.00000

etc.

15 BEST FEATURES ARE

FEATURE NAME	AVG. CORREL. COEFF.	MERIT VALUE
2MNT-3	0.53977	0.66803
SCS4	0.49439	0.62505
PO7-2	0.83549	0.62019
AREA	0.84854	0.61438
ARE-2	0.84854	0.61438
PO6-2	0.59520	0.58980
PO8-2	0.71349	0.52144
TPRB2	0.77316	0.51389
TPRB5	0.81658	0.51335
TPRB4	0.71853	0.46956
AVG-2	0.83089	0.44786
TPRB12	0.75441	0.44608
BIN3	0.75895	0.44579
SCS1-3	0.81971	0.43580
TPRB14	0.77637	0.43222

| AVERAGE --- | 0.74160 | |

by merging the two files for each feature. Feature values are ranked. A threshold is then moved through the ranked list starting at the low values, and the number of cells correctly classified at each setting of the threshold is constantly updated. If a feature value from the other data set is encountered, the threshold is temporarily set back. A tentative advance is made. If the value from the second data set is an outlier, and many more correct classifications could be gained by advancing the threshold, the single classification error is accepted. If, however, it becomes evident that advancement of the threshold would result in additional classification errors, the threshold is left at the original setting. The process is then repeated for the same feature starting at the high-value end of the ranked list and moving the threshold downward. This is repeated for every feature. The feature and the threshold setting which give the highest number of correct cell classifications are selected as the first feature and decision rule element. All cells thus classified are now removed from further consideration. The algorithm starts over again since the second best feature from the full data set may not be the best feature for the now reduced data set (Fig. 20).

The program lets the user specify how many of the best features should be used. It occurs frequently that a feature is selected repeatedly. The algorithm terminates when the next decision rule could not classify at least a chosen proportion of the as yet unclassified cells. This is necessary to avoid the setting of many thresholds, which only succeed in assigning individual cells in regions of the feature space where the two data sets overlap. Rather, such cells are left unclassified and the cells are thus labeled.

The DSELECT algorithm operates on the basis of a two category discrimination. It is a nonparametric procedure, i.e., it does not depend on any assumptions concerning the feature distributions. The algorithm has been in use for many years, and has proven itself stable, reliable, and not sensitive to particulars of data distributions. As an example, two sets of 198 Wright-stained images of human T cells and monocytes were submitted as training sets to the DSELECT algorithm. The decision sequence is shown in Table 10 and is to be evaluated as follows. The best feature is the cell area.

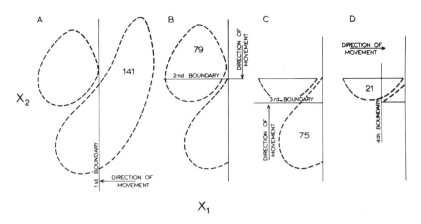

FIGURE 20. Schematic presentation of the algorithm DSELECT for a bivariate feature space. (A) Movement downward in value for feature X_1 produces correct classification for 141 points. These are classified and removed from further consideration. (B) Movement downward on the X_2 axis causes correct classification of 79 points. Process may continue as shown in (C) and (D).

TABLE 10
Results of DSELECT Algorithm Applied to Features of Human T Cells and Monocytes

STEP	CLASS[1]	DESCRIPTOR	THRESHOLD	POSITION[2]	NAME
1	2	3	749.000	1	AREA
2	1	15	0.192	-1	CND2
3	1	3	432.000	-1	AREA
4	1	1	0.151	-1	BIN2
5	2	3	690.000	1	AREA
6	1	11	146.260	1	MOMNT2
7	2	9	20.900	-1	POLR9
8	1	1	0.339	1	BIN2
9	2	5	424.000	1	ARN
10	1	1	0.302	1	BIN2
11	2	1	0.268	1	BIN2
12	1	11	72.282	-1	MOMNT2
13	2	4	32.171	1	AVG
14	1	6	34.232	1	AEN
15	2	1	0.214	-1	BIN2
16	1	1	0.244	-1	BIN2
17	2	1	0.244	1	BIN2

[1] 1 indicates T cells; 2 indicates B cells.
[2] -1 indicates position below the threshold; 1 indicates position above the threshold.

All cells with a relative cell area larger than 749 units are to be assigned to Group 2, i.e., to the monocyte category. The next best feature is a chromatin condensation index, CND2. All cell images with an index value of less than 0.192 are to be assigned to the T-cell category, and so forth.

The number of cells which are correctly classified, incorrectly classified, as well as those which could not be classified, and the classification errors are listed for each of the decision steps as shown below:

CLASS 1: T   CLASS 2: M

STEP	CLASS 1 (CORR)	CLASS 1 (ERROR)	CLASS 2 (CORR)	CLASS 2 (ERROR)
1	0	0	163	0
2	122	0	0	0
3	36	0	0	0
4	11	0	0	0
5	0	0	11	0
6	5	0	0	0
7	0	0	5	0
8	5	0	0	0
9	0	0	11	0
10	5	0	0	0
11	0	0	2	0
12	4	0	0	0
13	0	0	3	0
14	8	0	0	0
15	0	0	2	0
16	2	0	0	0
17	0	0	1	0

The printout also includes the following information:

0 POINTS IN CLASS 1 AND   0 POINTS IN CLASS 2 REMAIN UNCLASSIFIED.

198 POINTS ARE CLASSIFIED CORRECTLY AS BELONGING TO GROUP 1 PLUS   0 ERRORS.

198 POINTS ARE CLASSIFIED CORRECTLY AS BELONGING TO GROUP 2 PLUS   0 ERRORS.

ALPHA = 0.000   BETA = 0.000

As always, the decision rule is stored and applied to test set data. Test set data represent data for which the class membership is known and include data not used to derive the decision rule. The following shows the results obtained when the classification rule is applied to three different sets of T cells and three different sets of monocytes.

	T cells	Monocytes
T cells	97%	3%
	99%	1%
	99%	1%
Monocytes	7%	93%
	14%	86%
	1%	99%

2. Algorithm CLASFY

The second example is the algorithm CLASFY, by Cooley and Lohnes (1962). This requires a preselected set of features. It is a parametric procedure. The assumption is made that the feature values from each category follow multivariate normal distributions. The algorithm will allow many categories. Each may have a different mean vector and variance–covariance matrix for its feature values. In practice, one may use up to six categories and at most eight to ten features, although a lower number of features is preferable. The program estimates for each category the mean feature vector and the variance–covariance matrix. It then assigns each cell, on the basis of its feature vector, to the category with the maximum likelihood. The output provides the cell identification number, the assignment to a category, and the relative probabilities that a cell is a member of this or any other category. A sample run shows the options: One may "train" the algorithm and create a classification rule, or one may apply a previously generated decision rule to a test set of data. The printout shows a typical dialogue for the second option. The previously created decision rule had been stored as a file.

```
OPTIONS:
1 ——— CREATE DECISION RULE
2 ——— PROCEED WITH CLASSIFICATION
3 ——— EXIT
ENTER OPTION #: 2

ENTER INPUT DEVICE NAME<DP0,DK0,DK1>: DP0
 ACCEPT DEVICE "DP0": Y

WANT TO SAVE THE RESULT PRINTOUT: Y

YOUR SAVED PRINTOUT FILE "CLASIF.RST" IS ON SY0

ENTER SAVED DECISION RULE FILE NAME: M1317D
 ACCEPT: Y

IS TRUE CLASSIFICATION OF ITEMS IN FILE KNOWN: Y

ENTER NAME OF FILE TO BE CLASSIFIED: M135FB
WHICH GROUP ARE THOSE OBJECTS ASSUMED TO
     BELONG TO <1,2,3, . . . ,N>: 1
 ACCEPT: Y

 MORE DATA: N

ASSUMED GROUP # 1     TOTAL SAMPLE: 100

WANT TO SCALE THE DATA: N

USING EQUAL PRIOR PROBABILITIES FOR EACH GROUP: Y
```

The data represented lymphocytes from mice infected with leukemia virus and collected at certain times after infection. The training samples had been taken from control cells and a data set obtained from mice showing signs of infection and where every cell exhibited characteristics of virus-altered cells. The Group 1 represents control cells. A test is made to determine how many cells of a sample collected at a given time after the virus infection would still be classified as normal, unaltered cells. Presentation of the first 40 cells in Table 11 reveals that the majority of cells are classified as virus-altered cells. Since this was a test data set, only items supposedly being control cells were submitted. Only entries into row 1 of the classification table were made. The table shows that 92 of the 100 submitted cells were classified as showing an alteration.

CLASSIFICATION TABLE, ROWS ARE ACTUAL GROUPS, AND

COLUMNS ARE PREDICTED GROUPS

ROW 1	8	92
ROW 2	0	0

TABLE 11

Sample Printout of Data from CLASFY Algorithm for Murine Lymphocytes Obtained from Virus-Infected Animals

100 SUBJECTS		5 FEATURES	2 GROUPS
NAME		PR(1)	PR(2)
M135FB	1	0.0000	1.0000
M135FB	2	0.0028	0.9972
M135FB	3	0.1332	0.8668
M135FB	4	0.0000	1.0000
M135FB	5	0.0000	1.0000
M135FB	6	0.0000	1.0000
M135FB	7	0.0000	1.0000
M135FB	8	0.0000	1.0000
M135FB	9	0.0000	1.0000
M135FB	10	0.0000	1.0000
M135FB	11	0.0000	1.0000
M135FB	12	0.1949	0.8051
M135FB	13	0.0000	1.0000
M135FB	14	0.0428	0.9572
M135FB	15	0.0000	1.0000
M135FB	16	0.0000	1.0000
M135FB	17	0.0000	1.0000
M135FB	18	0.0000	1.0000
M135FB	19	0.0000	1.0000
M135FB	20	0.0000	1.0000
M135FB	21	0.0000	1.0000
M135FB	22	0.0000	1.0000
M135FB	23	1.0000	0.0000
M135FB	24	0.0000	1.0000
M135FB	25	0.9956	0.0044
M135FB	26	0.3970	0.6030
M135FB	27	0.0000	1.0000
M135FB	28	0.0000	1.0000
M135FB	29	0.0000	1.0000
M135FB	30	0.0713	0.9287
M135FB	31	0.0000	1.0000
M135FB	32	0.0000	1.0000
M135FB	33	0.0000	1.0000
M135FB	34	0.0000	1.0000
M135FB	35	0.5192	0.4808
M135FB	36	0.0000	1.0000
M135FB	37	0.0000	1.0000
M135FB	38	0.0000	1.0000
M135FB	39	0.0000	1.0000
M135FB	40	1.0000	0.0000
Etc.			

3. Discriminant Analysis

Multiple stepwise discriminant analysis is also a parametric procedure (Cooley and Lohnes, 1962). The assumption is that the variance–covariance matrices of all cell categories are the same. Even though the model is quite robust and violation of this assumption does in general not greatly affect the results, there are many instances in cell image analysis where gross deviations from the equality of the variance–covariance matrices occur, and where significant effects on the final result are exerted.

The multiple stepwise discriminant algorithm selects its own feature set in an incremental manner. Many programs, such as the BMD version (Dixon, 1967) and the SPSS version (Klecka *et al.*, 1975) offer options for the criterion used to add a feature to the selected subset. A frequently used criterion is Wilks' lambda (Cooley and Lohnes, 1962) which will be presented here. For information on the other options, the reader is referred to the SPSS program documentation.

Wilks' lambda is the multivariate analogon to the univariate F ratio. The F ratio is given by the ratio of two variances for a single feature. Wilks' lambda is formed similarly and is defined as the ratio of the determinant of the within groups variance–covariance matrix to the determinant of the total variance–covariance matrix. The determinant expresses the dispersion of a multivariate distribution. Wilks' lambda may range from zero to unity. A value of unity means that assignment of cells to categories has resulted in a dispersion of the classified data set which is equal to that of the unclassified data set; in other words, when Wilks' lambda = 1.00, there is no discrimination. A low value of Wilks' lambda means that the classification procedure has led to tightly formed groups, the dispersion of which is very small compared to that of the initial, unclassified data set. Features are sequentially selected so that Wilks' lambda is minimized. A sample run will be used to illustrate the operation of the program and the interpretation of results. First, the user may choose a criterion for feature selection:

ENTER NUMBER OF THE METHOD TO BE USED:
1. MINIMIZE WILKS' LAMBDA
2. MAXIMIZE MINIMUM MAHALANOBIS DISTANCE BETWEEN GROUP PAIRS
3. MAXIMIZE MINIMUM F BETWEEN GROUP PAIRS
4. MINIMIZE RESIDUAL UNEXPLAINED VARIATION
5. MAXIMIZE RAO'S V
6. DIRECT SOLUTION METHOD
METHOD? 1

He is then informed of some restrictions and asked to specify where his data are stored.

THE MAXIMUM NUMBER OF GROUPS THE PROGRAM CAN HANDLE IS 10.
PLEASE ENTER THE NUMBER OF GROUPS: 2

SELECT INPUT DEVICE:DPO,DK1,MTO:DPO

This is followed by some housekeeping chores, such as entering the file names and counts of the number of cells to be classified.

```
ENTER A 4 CHAR GROUP NAME FOR GROUP 1: M2T1
ENTER FILE NAME IN A6 <AAAAAA>: M2T100
THE GROUP SIZE IS: 126
```

GROUP COUNTS

GROUP 1 M2T1	GROUP 2 M2B1	TOTAL
126.0	126.0	

The means and standard deviations are printed out for the submitted feature set as shown in Table 12.

TABLE 12
Sample Printout of Group Means and Standard Deviations of Features from T and B Cells Submitted to Multiple Stepwise Discriminant Analysis

GROUP MEANS

	GROUP 1 M2T1	GROUP 2 M2B1
BIN3	0.2300	0.1042
BIN5	0.1386	0.1668
BIN7	0.0318	0.1218
ARE-2	1.2934	0.8840
TEE-4	0.3905	0.3883
AVG-2	0.3116	0.4457
PO6-2	0.2554	0.1526
PO7-2	0.1108	0.0140
PO8-2	0.0197	0.0002
2MNT-3	0.0231	0.0190
TPRB2	0.0614	0.0210
TPRB5	0.1433	0.0570
TPRB6	0.0156	0.0334
TPRB12	0.0207	0.0582
TPRB14	0.0233	0.0890
SCS1-3	0.3386	0.6319
SCS4	12.0992	7.1001

GROUP STANDARD DEVIATIONS

	GROUP 1 M2T1	GROUP 2 M2B1
BIN3	0.1038	0.0481
BIN5	0.0830	0.0582
BIN7	0.0383	0.0500
ARE-2	0.1755	0.1039
TEE-4	0.0443	0.0234
AVG-2	0.0754	0.0611
PO6-2	0.0391	0.0590
PO7-2	0.0401	0.0180
PO8-2	0.0193	0.0008
2MNT-3	0.0015	0.0016
TPRB2	0.0299	0.0126
TPRB5	0.0462	0.0339
TPRB6	0.0127	0.0107
TPRB12	0.0188	0.0195
TPRB14	0.0283	0.0344
SCS1-3	0.1486	0.1404
SCS4	1.8508	3.6007

The program next computes the within-cell-group variance–covariance matrix, averaged over all groups, and the overall or total variance–covariance matrix over all data points. The within-group correlation matrix shows which features are highly correlated (Table 13). The user is then requested to specify an F ratio for the inclusion of a variable in the finally selected feature set. For the sample sizes usually encountered in cell image analysis, i.e., from 100 to 250 cells per group, the number of features, and the number of groups, an F ratio of $F = 5.00$ leads to conservative classification results. When one has a favorable situation and large sample sizes with only two or three groups, an F ratio of $F = 3.00$ is still acceptable. An F ratio chosen lower than that, such as $F = 1.00$ may lead to the selection

TABLE 13

Sample Printout of Within-Group Correlation Matrix for T and B Cells Analyzed by Multiple Stepwise Discriminant Analysis

WITHIN GROUPS CORRELATION MATRIX

	BIN3[1]	BIN5	BIN7	ARE-2	TEE-4	AVG-2
BIN3	1.0000					
BIN5	-0.5513	1.0000				
BIN7	-0.5840	0.0548	1.0000			
ARE-2	0.7407	-0.3802	-0.6752	1.0000		
TEE-4	-0.7566	0.5516	0.5455	-0.6350	1.0000	
AVG-2	-0.7733	0.2920	0.7448	-0.9278	0.7630	1.0000
PO6-2	0.0787	0.4931	-0.3684	0.2824	0.2505	-0.3160
PO7-2	0.8051	-0.4196	-0.6433	0.8745	-0.6018	-0.7990
PO8-2	0.6500	-0.5954	-0.3914	0.7721	-0.6772	-0.6391
2MNT-3	-0.2439	0.4610	0.0669	0.0242	0.6747	0.1450
TPRB2	0.7006	-0.5784	-0.5257	0.8428	-0.7725	-0.8073
TPRB5	0.8205	-0.3819	-0.7256	0.8062	-0.7247	-0.8799
TPRB6	-0.4028	0.3487	0.4429	-0.5196	0.5542	0.5203
TPRB12	-0.5576	0.2480	0.4698	-0.6719	0.5940	0.7234
TPRB14	-0.6252	0.0593	0.8814	-0.7178	0.5991	0.8062
SCS1-3	-0.7576	0.1993	0.7372	-0.8656	0.7570	0.9711
SCS4	0.1034	-0.0635	0.0867	0.0048	-0.0979	-0.0078

	PO6-2	PO7-2	PO8-2	2MNT-3	TPRB2	TPRB5
PO6-2	1.0000					
PO7-2	0.2400	1.0000				
PO8-2	-0.2281	0.7205	1.0000			
2MNT-3	0.7326	0.0702	-0.2206	1.0000		
TPRB2	-0.1153	0.7024	0.8062	-0.3506	1.0000	
TPRB5	0.2486	0.8028	0.5363	-0.1878	0.7646	1.0000
TPRB6	0.0921	-0.4854	-0.4968	0.2834	-0.5168	-0.5030
TPRB12	-0.1981	-0.6150	-0.4704	0.1365	-0.6148	-0.7234
TPRB14	-0.3958	-0.6833	-0.4115	0.0702	-0.5614	-0.7760
SCS1-3	-0.3634	-0.7667	-0.5771	0.1331	-0.7353	-0.8633
SCS4	-0.0487	0.1077	0.0923	0.0001	0.0306	0.0287

	TPRB6	TPRB12	TPRB14	SCS1-3	SCS4	
TPRB6	1.0000					
TPRB12	0.6643	1.0000				
TPRB14	0.4195	0.5794	1.0000			
SCS1-3	0.4911	0.7376	0.8033	1.0000		
SCS4	0.0046	-0.0414	0.0148	-0.0517	1.0000	

[1]BIN and HIST are equivalent terms.

of a large number of features. The program may run for a long time, and there is a danger that variables are included which will not consistently discriminate. One may overtrain the classifier and obtain a classification rule which may prove to be ineffective once data not included in the training set are submitted for classification. One must also choose an option on prior probabilities of cells to fall into any of the groups.

PRIOR PROBABILITY OPTIONS
1. EQUAL
2. BASED ON GROUP SIZE
3. USER SPECIFIED
OPTION?: 2

PRIOR PROBABILITIES FOR GROUPS—
   M2T1   M2B1
  0.5000   0.5000

The stepwise discriminant procedure can now begin and an example is shown for the first few features (Table 14). One will notice that Wilks' lambda decreases as each variable is added. In this instance the first variable or feature, already leads to a Wilks' lambda of 0.29. This is unusual and indicates that excellent discrimination can be expected. It is more common to start with a Wilks' lambda of about 0.75 and to see it reduced to a value of 0.20 after 10–15 features have been chosen.

The significance of Wilks' lambda can be assessed from an F ratio with degrees of freedom determined by the number of features and the sample size minus the number of features plus one. In the example given here all the Wilks' lambda are highly significant at alpha smaller than 0.00001.

Then a significance test for the separation of group centroids is done:

THIS F RATIO IS THE SIGNIFICANCE TEST FOR THE MAHALANOBIS DISTANCE BETWEEN GROUP PAIRS. I.E., EQUALITY OF PAIRS OF CENTROIDS

F MATRIX—DEGREES OF FREEDOM: 11,   240
           GROUP 1
GROUP 2 139.43207

The algorithm, in this example, selected eleven features although it took fifteen steps (Table 15).

Since two cell categories were submitted, only one discriminant function will be formed. When, for example, three groups are submitted, two discriminant functions would have been formed. One is interested to see what relative proportion of the total information is retrieved by the first, the second, etc., discriminant functions; the program provides this information.

WILKS' LAMBDA HERE IS USED TO ASSESS STATISTICAL SIGNIFICANCE OF DISCRIMINA-
TION INFORMATION REMAINING. BEFORE ANY FUNCTION IS CONSIDERED, THE FULL
REDUCTION OF WILKS' LAMBDA ATTAINED BY ALL ENTERED VARIABLES APPLIES. WITH
THE FIRST DFCT EMPLOYED, LESS DISCRIMINATING INFO. REMAINS. ITS SIGNIFICANCE
IS EVALUATED BY A CHI-SQUARE TEST.

DFCT	EIGEN-VALUE	REL%	CANONICAL CORRELATION	FUNCT. DERIVED	WILKS' LAMBDA	CHI SQUARE	D.F.	SIGN.
				0	.13531	489.0525	11	.0000
1	6.39064	100.0	0.92989					

THE REMAINING COMPUTATIONS WILL BE BASED ON 1 DISCRIMINANT FUNCTIONS

TABLE 14
Sample Printout of the Stepwise Discriminant Procedure for Discrimination of Murine T and B Cells

VARIABLE ENTERED ON STEP 1:   PO7-2

				D.F.		SIGNIFICANCE
WILKS' LAMBDA	0.2899	APPROXIMATE F	612.387	1	250	.0000
RAO'S V	612.3886	CHANGE IN V	612.389	1		.0000

VARIABLE ENTERED ON STEP 2:   TEE-4

				D.F.		SIGNIFICANCE
WILKS' LAMBDA	0.2026	APPROXIMATE F	490.116	2	249	.0000
RAO'S V	984.2509	CHANGE IN V	371.862	1		.0000

VARIABLE ENTERED ON STEP 3:   SCS4

				D.F.		SIGNIFICANCE
WILKS' LAMBDA	0.1812	APPROXIMATE F	373.660	3	248	.0000
RAO'S V	1130.1144	CHANGE IN V	758.252	1		.0000

VARIABLE ENTERED ON STEP 4:   TPRB2

				D.F.		SIGNIFICANCE
WILKS' LAMBDA	0.1680	APPROXIMATE F	305.712	4	247	.0000
RAO'S V	1237.8981	CHANGE IN V	479.646	1		.0000

VARIABLE ENTERED ON STEP 5:   BIN7

				D.F.		SIGNIFICANCE
WILKS' LAMBDA	0.1596	APPROXIMATE F	259.075	4	246	.0000
RAO's V	1316.6404	CHANGE IN V	836.994	1		.0000

VARIABLE ENTERED ON STEP 6:   TPRB6

				D.F.		SIGNIFICANCE
WILKS' LAMBDA	0.1542	APPROXIMATE F	223.940	6	245	.0000
RAO'S V	1371.3385	CHANGE IN V	534.344	1		.0000

TABLE 15
Sample Printout of Summary Table for Multiple Stepwise Discriminant Analysis

SUMMARY TABLE
<E> FOR ENTERED; <R> FOR REMOVED

STEP NO.	VARIABLE	F TO ENTER OR REMOVE	NO. OF VAR.	WILK'S LAMBDA	SIGN.	RAO'S V	CHANGE IN RAO'S V	SIGN. OF CHANGE
1	E PO7-2	612.387	1	.28989	.0000	612.39	612.39	.0000
2	E TEE-4	107.346	2	.20257	.0000	984.25	371.86	.0000
3	E SCS4	29.308	3	.18116	.0000	1742.50	758.25	.0000
4	E TPRB2	19.273	4	.16804	.0000	2222.15	479.65	.0000
5	E BIN7	13.020	5	.15960	.0000	3059.14	836.99	.0000
6	E TPRB6	8.543	6	.15422	.0000	3593.49	534.34	.0000
7	E SCS1-3	4.155	7	.15164	.0000	4458.10	864.62	.0000
8	R BIN7	3.633	6	.15390	.0000	4968.26	510.16	.0000
9	E AVE-2	8.612	7	.14865	.0000	5889.73	921.47	.0000
10	E TPRB14	6.481	8	.14479	.0000	6444.71	554.97	.0000
11	E BIN5	6.230	9	.14115	.0000	7410.61	965.91	.0000
12	E PO6-2	6.080	10	.13768	.0000	8010.38	599.77	.0000
13	E PO8-2	4.196	11	.13531	.0000	9009.28	997.90	.0000
14	R PO8-2	4.196	10	.13768	.0000	9576.05	567.78	.0000
15	E PO8-2	4.196	11	.13531	.0000	10605.94	1029.89	.0000

STANDARDIZED DISCRIMINANT
FUNCTION COEFFICIENTS

	DFCT 1
BIN5	-0.1125
TEE-4	0.6926
AVG-2	0.5950
PO6-2	-0.2808
PO7-2	0.3965
PO8-2	-0.1348
TPRB2	0.2601
TPRB6	-0.1171
TPRB14	-0.2460
SCS1-3	-1.0004
SCS4	0.1729

UNSTANDARDIZED DISCRIMINANT
FUNCTION COEFFICIENTS

	DFCT 1
BIN5	-1.5429
TEE-4	19.5984
AVG-2	6.2036
PO6-2	-3.9140
PO7-2	6.8853
PO8-2	-8.0399
TPRB2	8.5089
TPRB6	-7.9461
TPRB14	-5.4029
SCS1-3	-4.8577
SCS4	0.0455
CONST.	-7.2279

If the eigenvalue associated with the last discriminant function forms only a fraction of a percent of the trace, then the function simply does not convey much information and may be totally insignificant. The standardized discriminant function coefficients, in their absolute values, reflect the relative contribution that each feature makes to the discrimination (see the bottom part of Table 15).

The unstandardized discriminant function coefficients are the actual weights used to compute for each cell feature vector its position on the discriminant axis.

The final classification results are presented as follows:

1. A list of the cell ID and its actual cell category.
2. The category for which the probability of membership was highest, i.e., the classification result for that cell.
3. Column $P(X|G)$ lists the probability to obtain a value for the discriminant function as found in this cell, given that it was a member of that cell category. This is in a way a measure of how typical the cell is for its own class.
4. The next column lists the probability $P(G|X)$ that the cell is a member of that cell category, given that a value X for the discriminant function had been found.
5. This information is also provided for the cell category with the next highest probability.

Finally, the discriminant function value for the cell is printed out as shown below. Classification errors are flagged by a series of asterisks.

CASE FILE	ACTUAL			HIGHEST PROBABILITY			2ND HIGHEST		DISCRIMINANT
	SEQ	GROUP		GROUP	P (X/G)	P (G/X)	GROUP	P (G/X)	DFCT 1
M2T100	1	1		1	1.000	1.000			0.572
M2T100	2	1		1	0.963	0.911	2	0.089	
M2T100	3	1		1	1.000	1.000			0.907
M2T100	4	1		1	1.000	1.000			1.100
M2T100	5	1		1	1.000	1.000			1.250
M2T100	6	1		1	1.000	1.000			1.236
M2T100	7	1		1	1.000	1.000			0.711
M2T100	8	1		1	1.000	1.000			0.798
M2T100	9	1		1	1.000	1.000			0.700
etc.									
M2B100	78	2		2	1.000	1.000			−0.866
M2B100	79	2		2	1.000	1.000			−0.661
M2B100	80	2	****	1	0.961	0.906			−0.166

Finally, a confusion matrix is printed out.

PREDICTION RESULTS—

ACTUAL GROUP	NO. OF CASES	PREDICTED GROUP MEMBERSHIP	
		GP. 1	GP. 2
GROUP 1	126	125	1
M2T1		99.2%	0.8%
GROUP 2	126	3	123
M2B1		2.4%	97.6%

PERCENT OF "GROUPED" CASES CORRECTLY CLASSIFIED: 98.41%

E. Unsupervised Learning Algorithms

Unsupervised learning algorithms accept a data set of feature vectors and attempt to partition it into two or more subsets. If the ensuing subsets can be proven to be statistically significantly different, one has detected "modes" in the feature space which indicate an inhomogeneity of the feature vectors or among the cell images which they represent. The unsupervised learning techniques are important tools because the detection may be based solely on the structure of the data in feature space and the inhomogeneity of a cell population may not have been apparent to visual inspection.

1. Feature Selection for Unsupervised Learning

If one does not know if a cell population contains subsets of cells, one really has no definite clues as to which features might be suitable to detect the subsets. An added difficulty is that unsupervised learning algorithms usually require substantial core, and one is therefore restricted in the number of features which one can combine to form feature vectors. As a rule it is impractical on a laboratory computer to consider a clustering procedure on a data set of more than 10-dimensional feature vectors. A dimensionality of 4–6 is much more common.

Nevertheless, the selection of suitable features may follow some guidelines. If there are subsets of feature vectors, and they are separated into modes in feature space, one may assume that the direction of greatest variance of the entire data set is determined by those features that separate the subsets. Therefore, if one computes the principal components, the features with the greatest coefficients are a good choice as features for unsupervised learning. This is demonstrated for a combined data set of mouse B and T cells. Figure 21 shows a plot of the first principal component, i.e., of the direction of greatest variance. The inhomogeneity is clearly indicated. One may also make an educated guess and look for subsets of T cells

```
RANGE   PERCENT TOTAL        FILE: M2TB10     FEATURE: PRNCM1
0.000     6.75  ( 17) I*********************************
0.050     5.95  ( 15) I*****************************
0.100     9.92  ( 25) I*************************************************
0.150     9.13  ( 23) I*********************************************
0.200     6.35  ( 16) I*******************************
0.250     7.54  ( 19) I*************************************
0.300     1.98  (  5) I********
0.350     3.57  (  9) I*****************
0.400     4.37  ( 11) I*********************
0.450     4.37  ( 11) I*********************
0.500     3.57  (  9) I*****************
0.550     5.95  ( 15) I*****************************
0.600     4.76  ( 12) I***********************
0.650     3.57  (  9) I*****************
0.700     3.97  ( 10) I*******************
0.750     1.98  (  5) I********
0.800     2.38  (  6) I**********
0.850     3.57  (  9) I*****************
0.900     3.97  ( 10) I*******************
0.950     0.79  (  2) I*
1.000     5.56  ( 14) I***************************
```

FIGURE 21. Computer printout of a distribution of values of the first principal component for T and B cells.

by using the feature set which maximally separates B and T cells. Finally, one may employ a brute force technique. Small subsets of features are tried, until a significant partitioning is established. The formed groups are submitted as training sets to a supervised learning algorithm. These algorithms quickly identify which other features separate the subsets. The features are now retrieved and submitted to the unsupervised learning algorithm.

2. The Basic KMEANS Algorithm

This algorithm starts by computing the mean feature vector for the entire data set (Duda and Hart, 1973). A random-number generator is then called, and two values are generated which perturb the mean. These two points in feature space serve as initial cluster centroids. Every feature vector is now assigned to the initial centroid to which it is nearest by some distance measure, typically by Euclidean distance. These assignments result in two subsets. For each, a new centroid is computed. As a rule the shift in centroids results in several reassignments of points from one cluster to another, and *vice versa*. This process is repeated until no reassignments occur after a recomputation of the mean values. The grouping procedure has converged. If one is searching for a partitioning into more than two subsets, the random-number generator is set to generate as many perturbed, initial cluster centroids as the number of subsets one suspects might be present. Usually one does not know how many there might be. The program simply is set to form two subsets, and then three, four, etc., until a specified number is reached.

After the algorithm has converged, one will try to test for the significance of differences between subsets. A test statistic which has proven very useful is Beale's test statistic. It compares the sum of squares of all deviations from the multivariate mean which one obtains with a grouping into, for example, two subsets to that of the undivided data set. If the grouping leads to a lower sum of squares, the feature space may indeed have two modes. In an analogous fashion one may test whether a partitioning into, for example, four subsets is a better fit to the data than a grouping into fewer subsets.

Beale's test statistic (Beale, 1969) computes as

$$F(c_i,c_j) = \frac{\text{RVAL}_{c_i} - \text{RVAL}_{c_j}}{\text{RVAL}_{c_j}} \bigg/ \left\{ \frac{n-c_i}{n-c_j} \left(\frac{c_j}{c_i}\right)^{2/p} - 1 \right\}$$

and is distributed as an F ratio with $p(c_j-c_i)$ and $p(n-c_j)$ degrees of freedom. In this equation, RVAL_{c_j} stands for the sum of squares obtained from j subsets, and RVAL_{c_i} stands for that obtained from i subsets; $c_j>c_i$; n is the number of feature vectors, and p stands for their dimensionality.

3. The PINDEX Algorithm

The PINDEX algorithm (McClellan, 1971) adds a refinement to this grouping procedure. When the grouping has converged, and subsets have been formed, the variance–covariance matrices of the formed subsets are computed. Reassignments are now made on the basis of maximum likelihood. This amounts to the use of a distance metric which is adaptive to the "shape" of the emerging clusters. Reassignments are made until convergence occurs. Then mean and covariance matrices are recomputed and the necessary reassignments are made. This is repeated until complete convergence has been achieved. The PINDEX algorithm is very useful, but not as robust as the KMEANS algorithm. For example, if a group is formed which contains fewer members than the feature space has dimensions, the eigenvalues of the covariance matrix go to zero, and the grouping stops. The process is illustrated with a sample run. In this run two data sets of known categories had been merged, to test the performance of the grouping procedure. The data were a merged file of mouse lymphocytes, 100 control cells, and 100 cells from a virus-infected animal. Five features had been chosen. The algorithm first computes the mean vector for the entire data set and the sum of squares about the mean (RVAL); the latter is required for Beale's test statistic later on.

THE CENTROID OF CLUSTER 1 IS
0.07056   0.06455   0.40396   0.61182   0.1671

MODE   1
        200

RVAL (1) = 21.7188

WANT TO SAVE GROUPED CELL ID: Y
ENTER SAVED GROUPED FILE NAME: MCELL ACCEPT: Y
...... SEARCH FOR 2 CLUSTER

USE ADAPTIVE DISTANCE MEASURE

THE INITIAL CLUSTER CENTROIDS ARE

MODE	1	2	3	4	5
1	0.072	0.078	0.404	0.701	0.018
2	0.074	0.085	0.449	0.697	0.019

98 RECLASSIFICATIONS THIS CYCLE
4 RECLASSIFICATIONS THIS CYCLE
NO CLASSIFICATION CHANGES

DISTANCE MEASURE REDEFINED

1 RECLASSIFICATION THIS CYCLE
NO CLASSIFICATION CHANGES

FINAL CLASSIFICATION IS

1	2	3	4	5	6	7	8	9	10	11	12	13	14	15	16	17	18
:	:	:	:	:	:	:	:	:	:	:	:	:	:	:	:	:	:
1	1	1	1	1	1	1	1	1	1	1	1	1	1	2	1	1	2

19	20	21	22	23	24	25	26	27	28	29	30	31	32	33	34	35	36
:	:	:	:	:	:	:	:	:	:	:	:	:	:	:	:	:	:
1	1	1	1	1	1	1	1	1	1	1	1	1	1	1	1	1	1

The assignment to either of two groups is shown for the first 36 feature vectors. The control cells and the altered cells have rather different characteristics, the algorithm therefore converges rather rapidly.

THE CENTROID OF CLUSTER 1 IS
0.02484   0.00337   0.26497   0.36069   0.00244

THE CENTROID OF CLUSTER 2 IS
0.11362   0.12216   0.53484   0.84831   0.03016

MODE   1   2
        97   103

RVAL (2) = 5.0655

One can see that the unsupervised grouping procedure divides the data set into two groups of approximately equal size. This agrees in fact with the true cell classification which was known in this case. The sum of squares for a partitioning of the data set into two groups is markedly reduced compared to the sum of squares computed for the entire data set.

The program finally inquires whether the assignment should be stored for each cell. Then the results from Beale's significance test are printed out. In this case, the null hypothesis can be rejected at an alpha level of less than 0.01, i.e., the two formed subgroups are statistically significant.

WANT TO SAVE GROUPED CELL ID: N

TRIAL GROUPING	# GROUPS COMPARISON	DEGREES OF FREEDOM		F-RATIO	ALPHA LEVEL
2	1	5	990	10.079	0.00%

The value of the test statistic, $F = 10.079$, is obtained as follows, for the data here:

$$F = \frac{21.7188 - 5.0655}{5.0655} \bigg/ \left[\frac{200 - 1}{200 - 2} \left(\frac{2}{1}\right)^{2/5} - 1 \right]$$
$$= 3.287592 \bigg/ \frac{199}{198} \times 2^{2/5} - 1$$
$$= 3.287592 / 1.00505 \times 1.3195 - 1$$
$$= 3.287592 / 0.326172$$

The value of the term $(c_j/c_i)^{2/p}$ is found by taking the log of c_j/c_i, multiplying the log by a factor of 2, dividing by p, and taking the antilog.

The grouping does not always converge as rapidly: The following sample run demonstrates a situation where the algorithm encounters several problems (Table 16). The algorithm here was instructed to try to form four groups. One of the randomly generated starting centroids, however, received no assignments. Later, the second eigenvalue of a group's variance–covariance matrix goes to zero as a recomputation is made—which the program announces with the printout "distance measure redefined." The algorithm stops. The groups for which the eigenvalue has gone to zero

TABLE 16
Sample Printout of PINDEX Algorithm

```
RVAL( 3)=     1.9677

WANT TO SAVE GROUPED CELL ID:  N
...... SEARCH FOR   4 CLUSTERS
USE ADAPTIVE DISTANCE MEASURE

              THE INITIAL CLUSTER CENTROIDS ARE
MODE       1       2       3       4       5
    1    0.078   0.089   0.443   0.702   0.019
    2    0.092   0.085   0.432   0.676   0.019
    3    0.089   0.072   0.444   0.697   0.019
    4    0.078   0.075   0.445   0.644   0.018
           167 RECLASSIFICATIONS THIS CYCLE
             3 HAS NO MEMBERS
             3 HAS NO MEMBERS
             3 HAS NO MEMBERS
             3 HAS NO MEMBERS
             3 HAS NO MEMBERS
            26 RECLASSIFICATIONS THIS CYCLE
            36 RECLASSIFICATIONS THIS CYCLE
             7 RECLASSIFICATIONS THIS CYCLE
             2 RECLASSIFICATIONS THIS CYCLE
             1 RECLASSIFICATIONS THIS CYCLE
          NO CLASSIFICATION CHANGES

          DISTANCE MEASURE REDEFINED

             5 RECLASSIFICATIONS THIS CYCLE
             "ETC"

            12 RECLASSIFICATIONS THIS CYCLE
             1 RECLASSIFICATIONS THIS CYCLE
          NO CLASSIFICATION CHANGES

          DISTANCE MEASURE REDEFINED

            13 RECLASSIFICATIONS THIS CYCLE
             5 RECLASSIFICATIONS THIS CYCLE
             2 RECLASSIFICATIONS THIS CYCLE
          NO CLASSIFICATION CHANGES

             2 EIGENVALUE GONE TO ZERO
GROUP HAS BEEN FORMED WITH FEWER MEMBERS THAN THE NUMBER OF FEATURES USED
FINAL CLASSIFICATION IS
 1  2  3  4  5  6  7  8  9  10  11  12  13  14  15  16  17  18
 :  :  :  :  :  :  :  :  :   :   :   :   :   :   :   :   :   :
 2  2  2  2  2  2  4  4  4   4   4   4   4   2   2   2   2   2
```

received fewer assignments than features had been used. The algorithm stops and merely lists the assignments made up to that point.

V. APPLICATION OF IMAGE ANALYSIS TO BIOLOGICAL PROBLEMS

Image analysis has been applied to lymphoid cells obtained from various species and subjected to different physical, biological, and chemical assaults. These studies are summarized in Table 17. The value of image

TABLE 17

Summary of Some of the Studies Concerned with the Analysis of Lymphocytes by Microphotometric Means

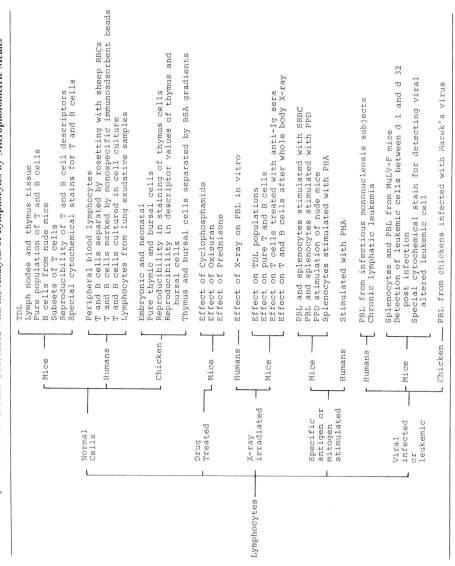

Lymphocytes

Normal Cells

Mice
- TDL
- Lymph nodes and thymus tissue
- Pure population of T and B cells
- B cells from nude mice
- Subsets of T cells
- Reproducibility of T and B cell descriptors
- Special cytochemical stains for T and B cells

Humans
- Peripheral blood lymphocytes
- T and B cells separated by rosetting with sheep RBCs
- T and B cells marked by monospecific immunoadsorbent beads
- T and B cells cultured in cell culture
- Lymphocytes from lung exudative samples

Chicken
- Embryonic and neonatal
- Pure thymic and bursal cells
- Reproducibility in staining of thymus cells
- Reproducibility in descriptor values of thymus and bursal cells
- Thymus and bursal cells separated by BSA gradients

Drug Treated

Mice
- Effect of Cyclophosphamide
- Effect of Oxisuran
- Effect of Prednisone

X-ray irradiated

Humans
- Effect of X-ray on PBL in vitro

Mice
- Effect on TDL populations
- Effect on pure T and B cells
- Effect on T cells treated with anti-Ig sera
- Effect on T and B cells after whole body X-ray

Specific antigen or mitogen stimulated

Mice
- PBL and splenocytes stimulated with SRBC
- PBL and splenocytes stimulated with PPD
- PPD stimulation of nude mice
- Splenocytes stimulated with PHA

Humans
- Stimulated with PHA

Viral infected or leukemic

Humans
- PBL from infectious mononucleosis subjects
- Chronic lymphatic leukemia

Mice
- Splenocytes and PBL from MuLV-F mice
- Detection of leukemic cells between d 1 and d 32 post infection
- Special cytochemical stain for detecting viral altered leukemic cell

Chicken
- PBL from chickens infected with Marek's virus

analytical methods to understanding and gaining additional information from biologic studies can be demonstrated by viewing the application of these analyses to lymphoid cells obtained from X-ray irradiated cell populations, virus-infected animals, and in the differentiation of lymphoid cells into subpopulations of cells.

A. X-Ray Radiation: Study One

Thoracic duct lymphocytes (TDL) were obtained from CBA mice by cannulation of the thoracic duct (Olson *et al.,* 1974). The relative numbers of T and B cells were determined using a fluorescein labeled polyvalent anti-Ig as a B-cell marker and the trypan blue exclusion test using rabbit anti-mouse-brain theta serum and complement as a T-cell marker (Boak and Woodruff, 1965). Other portions of cells suspended in minimum essential media with 10% fetal calf serum at a concentration of 5×10^6 cells/ml were irradiated at room temperature in uniform fashion utilizing a General Electric X-ray machine (120 kV peak, 15 mA, HLV 2.3 mm Cu, Thoraeus filter) (Anderson *et al.,* 1975b). The absorbed dose rate was 99 rads/min at 26 cm. Cells received doses ranging from 50 to 2000 rads. Immediately after irradiation, the cells were centrifuged at room temperature for 10 min at 1200 rpm and then resuspended in 0.25 ml of medium. The cell suspension was applied immediately to clean microscope slides, air dried, and fixed with 90% methanol and 10% acetic acid. The slides were hydrated, and the cells hydrolyzed in 5 N HCl for 20 min, stained with Schiff reagent for 2 h at room temperature, immersed three times in 5% (v/v) sulfurous acid for a total of 6 min, washed in tap water for 10 min, and dehydrated (Anderson *et al.,* 1975b; Deitch, 1966).

One hundred or more cells from each slide were scanned at a scanning spot size of 0.5×0.5 μm^2 and the data recorded as described in the first portion of this chapter.

Analysis of TDL subjected to 0, 50, 100, 500, and 2000 rads using some of the features and analytical programs described earlier show the following. The distribution of OD values of Feulgen-positive nuclear DNA appears to depend upon the amount of radiation the cells received. Figure 22 shows small to moderate amounts (50–100 rads) of radiation to cause a shift toward lower OD values. A reversal of this trend is experienced in cells exposed to 2000 rads where a marked spreading of OD values and increased proportion of high OD values are evident. The total amount of Feulgen-positive DNA and relative nuclear area of the cells demonstrate very little change as assessed by an analysis of variance of the data (Table 18).

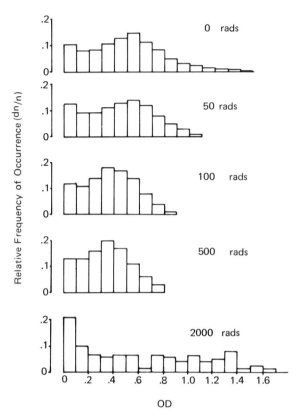

FIGURE 22. Distribution of optical density values from Feulgen-stained murine thoracic-duct lymphocytes exposed to various doses of X-ray irradiation.

These features reflect quantitative measurements of changes which can be visually detected in the cells. Cells exposed to 100 and 500 rads show increasing numbers of intranuclear vacuoles whereas the cells exposed to 2000 rads possess slightly smaller and pycnotic nuclei with no detectable intranuclear vacuoles.

An analysis of individual cells of the 0 rad group showed that 27% had high OD values (greater than 1.000 units) while 73% had OD values of a lesser magnitude. This percentage was comparable to the number of B cells in the population and raised the question whether this might be a feature to differentiate T and B cells. To investigate this possibility, we checked for features other than relative nuclear area, total optical density, and relative frequency of OD values to determine if there were other features which

TABLE 18

Total Optical Density and Relative Nuclear Area of Thoracic Duct
Lymphocytes Exposed to Various Doses of X-Ray Irradiation

Radiation dose (rads)	Total OD[a]	Relative nuclear area
0	4937	99.6
50	5161	112.6
100	4145	110.9
500	4024	114.3
2000	4505	98.5
$CL_{95}\%$ [b]	±71	±4.1

[a]Results are expressed as the number of 0.5×0.5 μm^2 OD readings per nucleus for relative nuclear area and the sum of the values of OD readings per nucleus for total OD.

[b]$CL_{95}\%$ = confidence limits expressed at 95% level. Computed on the mean square error term of the analysis of variance table.

would differentiate this smaller group of cells. Comparison showed HIST 4 (0.31–4.0 OD) and HIST 5 (0.41–0.50 OD) to be significant. Figure 23 shows a bivariate distribution of HIST 4 vs. HIST 5 of 0 rad TDL for cells with extended histograms (dense granules) and for cells with less dense granules. The figure shows that the cells with dense granules form a subpopulation which is grouped in the lower left corner. A regression line (discriminant 1) can be fitted through the data points and a distribution plot showing the percentage of cells falling into these two groups can be superimposed on the bivariate plot. A bimodal distribution is apparent and we arbitrarily refer to the small cell population as Mode 1 and to the larger population as Mode 2.

B cells are considered to be more radiosensitive than T cells (Anderson et al., 1977). We extended the logic that if Mode 1 represented B cells, these cells should display greater change to irradiation. Data on relative nuclear area, total OD, and relative frequency of OD values suggest the greatest damage occurred in cells irradiated at 500 rads. Figure 24 shows a bivariate plot of HIST 4 and HIST 5 for cells given 500 rads. A bimodal distribution in which 75% of the cells (Mode 2) comprise one mode and 25% a second mode (Mode 3) is evident. The larger mode appears to be relatively unchanged. This can be documented by creating subfiles of cells comprising the cells depicted in the modes of Fig. 23 and Fig. 24 and determining the histograms of OD values for the cell populations. Figure 25 shows that in each case, the histograms of Mode 2 remain unchanged whereas the histogram of Mode 1 (0 rad) disappears and is apparently replaced by the

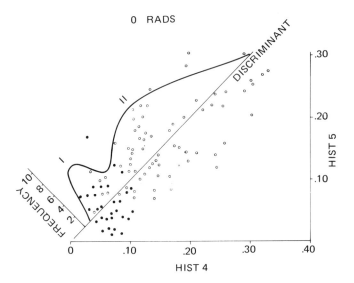

FIGURE 23. Bivariate plot of HIST 4, HIST 5 from Feulgen-stained nonirradiated thoracic-duct lymphocytes from CBA mice. Closed circles represent cell images with dense stained granules; open circles represent cell images with less dense granules. Figure also shows frequency distribution of these two cell populations.

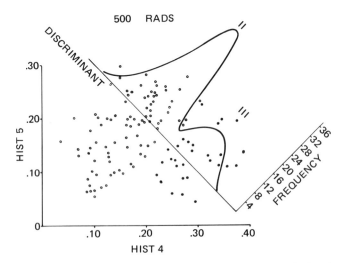

FIGURE 24. Bivariate plot of HIST 4, HIST 5 from Feulgen-stained thoracic-duct lymphocytes exposed to 500-rad radiation *in vitro*. Closed circles represent cell images with dense stained granules; open circles represent cell images with less dense granules. Figure shows frequency distribution of these two cell populations.

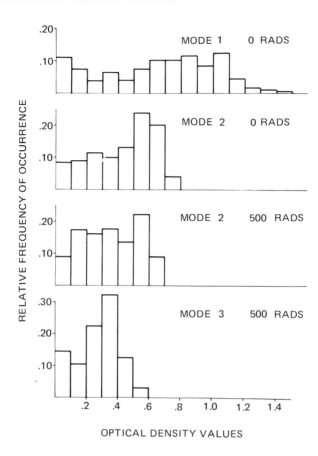

FIGURE 25. Distribution of optical density values from Feulgen-stained thoracic-duct lymphocytes exposed to 0- and 500-rad radiation *in vitro*. Mode two represents cell images shown in open circles on Figs. 23 and 24. Mode one represents cell images with closed circles on Fig. 23. Mode three represents cell images with closed circles on Fig. 24.

shorter histogram of Mode 3 (500 rads). The relationship of this shift in histograms is comparable to that observed in the entire TDL population subjected to 50–500 rads of irradiation.

To ascertain if the hypothesis that Mode 1 and Mode 3 represent a more radiosensitive B-cell population is a valid one, we conducted Study Two (Anderson *et al.*, 1975a).

B. X-Ray Radiation: Study Two

TDL were obtained from CBA and congenitally athymic (nu/nu) mice during the initial 10 h of cannulation of the thoracic duct (Boak and Woodruff, 1965). TDL from CBA were treated with previously absorbed poly-valent anti-Ig plus heat-inactivated absorbed guinea pig complement to destroy all B cells. The resultant cell suspension failed to respond to lipo-polysaccharide mitogens but did respond to phytohemagglutinin. Cells were suspended, irradiated and stained as described in Study One (Ander-son *et al.*, 1975). One hundred twenty-six cells from each slide were scanned and analyzed.

Analysis of B and T cells subjected to 0, 50, 100, and 2000 rads using the same features described earlier showed the following. The distribution of OD values of Feulgen-positive nuclear DNA in B cells showed a definite shift toward lighter-staining granules. The distribution of OD values of T cells showed no change for cells given 50 and 100 rads and a shift toward denser granules in cells exposed to 2000 rads (Fig. 26). Analysis also revealed a significant dose-dependent increase in relative nuclear area for B cells, which was not detected in T cells. Inspection of the nuclei of both cell populations depicted increasing vacuolization as a function of radiation dose in B cells. T cells given 2000 rads possessed densely stained pycnotic nuclei.

Similar experiments have detected radiation induced changes in lym-phoid cells in doses as small as 5 rads. These data demonstrate the value of image analysis as an investigative technique in detecting minute changes in cells subjected to such environmental physical events as irradiation.

C. X-Ray Radiation: Study Three

The purpose of this study was (a) to determine the relative radiosensi-tivity of human T and B cells of peripheral blood irradiated *in vitro* and (b) to ascertain whether image analysis could detect differences in the irradi-ated and nonirradiated cells which could be correlated to such biologic descriptors as cell viability, relative numbers of T and B cells as detected by immunofluorescence, and responsiveness of cells to mitogenic stimulation.

Peripheral blood lymphocytes (PBL) were obtained from two healthy adult male donors at yearly intervals over a three-year period. In each case the PBL were separated from defibrinated blood by centrifugation on a Ficoll–Hypaque gradient (Bozum, 1968). The cells were washed and sus-pended in minimum essential medium with 15% fetal calf serum. Each cell suspension was divided into four equal parts and subjected to 0, 5, 50, and 500 rads of radiation as described earlier. Irradiated cells were (a) cultured *in vitro* with different concentrations of concanavalin A (Con A) and phy-tohemagglutinin (PHA), (b) placed directly on microscope slides and

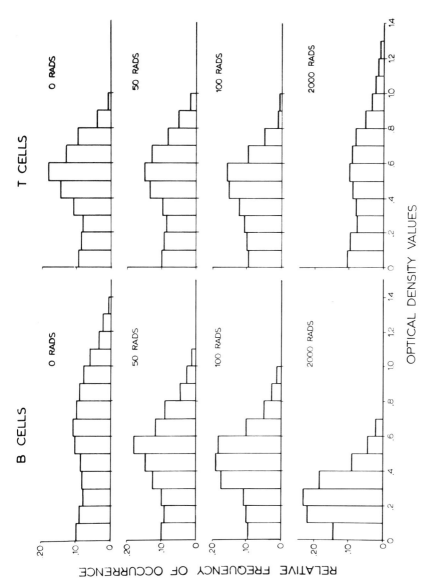

FIGURE 26. Distribution of optical density values from Feulgen-stained purified murine T and B cells exposed to various doses of X-ray irradiation.

stained for scanning, and (c) placed into culture tubes to determine changes in viability and survival of irradiated T and B cells during the subsequent 72 h.

In each of the three studies, results were very similar and can be represented by data from the final experiment. In nonirradiated cells, at time zero, the percentage of T and B cells for subject one was 75% T and 25% B and for subject two it was 78% T, 18% B, and 4% nonfluorescence-tagged cells. Figure 27 presents data to show that for both cell types and both subjects, a progressive loss of viability occurs with time among nonirradiated lymphocytes. With irradiation, in general, this loss is (a) more pronounced, (b) dose dependent, (c) time related and (d) greater for B than T cells. There are, however, differences between the two subjects: (a) the T cells of subject one appear to be more radiosensitive than the T cells of subject two, and (b) conversely, the B cells of subject two are more radiosensitive than those of subject one.

Additional differences in the biologic descriptors became apparent when a comparison of irradiation upon the responsiveness of PBL to PHA and Con A was made. Nonirradiated cells of subject one were more responsive to PHA stimulation than were the cells of subject two. Both subjects responded equally to Con A. This is reflected in the PHA:Con A ratios presented in Fig. 28. The greater PHA:Con A ratio of subject one continued to increase when the cells were exposed to 5 and 50 rads but returned to

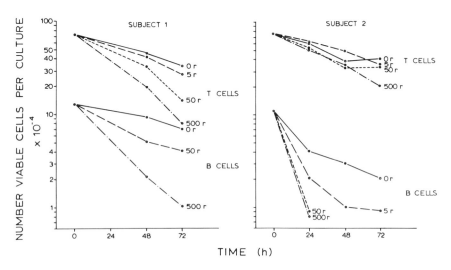

FIGURE 27. Viability of T and B cells from human subjects when cultured *in vitro* after exposure to various doses of X-ray irradiation.

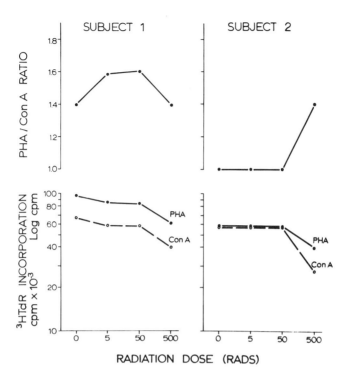

FIGURE 28. Degree of ³HTdR incorporation and PHA:Con A mitogen stimulation ratio for human lymphocytes when cultured *in vitro* after exposure to various doses of X-ray irradiation.

near control values following 500 rads of exposure (Stobo and Paul, 1973). The ratio of subject two remained at 1.0 until after the cells were exposed to 500 rads at which time the ratio increased to 1.4 (Olsen *et al.,* 1979a).

Relative nuclear area and total OD of cells showed consistent differences dependent upon the radiation dose and subject (Table 19). Cells of subject one reflect a dose-related increase in both relative nuclear area and total OD while cells of subject two show little if any change in these two descriptors. The same trend is observed in an analysis of the relative frequency of OD values of the Feulgen-stained DNA (Fig. 29). Subject two appears stable while the OD values of lymphocytes from subject one show a dose-related shift toward less dense Feulgen-positive DNA. It should be noted that the nonirradiated cells of subject one contained denser-stained granules of Feulgen-positive DNA than did the cells of subject two.

The dose-dependent effect of irradiation on relative nuclear area can

TABLE 19
**Total Optical Density and Relative Nuclear Area of Human
Lymphocytes Exposed to Various Levels of X-Ray Irradiation**

| Radiation dose | Total OD[a] | | Relative nuclear area | |
(rads)	Subject 1	Subject[b]	Subject 1	Subject 2
0	5595	5575	119	157
5	5437	5792	115	165
50	6171	5501	161	152
500	6210	5556	167	150
$CL_{95}\%^2$	±25	±25	±3	±3

[a]Results are expressed as the number of $0.5 \times 0.5\ \mu m^2$ OD per nucleus
for relative nuclear area and the sum of the value of OD readings per
nucleus for total OD.
[b]$CL_{95}\%$ = confidence limits expressed at the 95% level. Computed on the
mean square error term of the analysis of variance table.

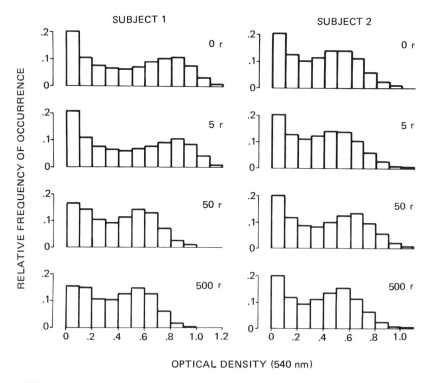

OPTICAL DENSITY (540 nm)

FIGURE 29. Distribution of optical density values from Feulgen-stained lymphocytes of
human subjects exposed to various doses of X-ray irradiation.

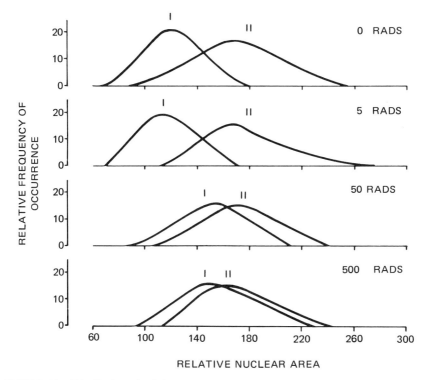

FIGURE 30. Distribution of cell images as a function of relative nuclear area of Feulgen-stained lymphocytes from two subjects exposed to various doses of X-ray irradiation *in vitro*.

be observed better in Fig. 30 which shows that the bimodal distribution created by the cell populations of the two subjects disappears as a function of radiation dose. At 500 rads the cells of subject one appear to overlap those of subject two (mean of 167 ± 25 and 150 ± 25, respectively).

A search in nonirradiated and irradiated cells of both subjects for other features with high discriminatory value can be made using the AMBIGUITY FUNCTION and FMERIT FUNCTION programs as described earlier. Submitting a selection of 10 features out of a possible 150 to a multiple stepwise discriminant analysis results in a further selection and ranking of the features most important for discrimination of nonirradiated from irradiated cells. These are average OD, radial OD profile values located $1.0-1.5\mu$m from the center of the nucleus, transition probabilities of OD values for the OD range of $0.41-0.60$ to $0.81-1.0$, and an index of chromatin heterogeneity as determined by one of the OD mesh texture analysis programs. Data obtained from such an analysis of cells may be plotted as frequency of occurrence vs the value of the discriminant function (Fig. 31). Comparison of irradiated and nonirradiated cells of subject two show little difference. Correct classification ranges from 57% when comparing nonirradiated cells to cells given 5 rads to 74% with cells exposed to 500 rads. The radiosensitivity of cells of subject one is apparent as discrimination success of 90 and 99% is observed for cells exposed to 50 and 500 rads (a discrimination success of 100% indicates no overlap between the two populations).

Both biologic and analytical data support the idea that the distributions of PBL in the two subjects are different and that the cells with the smaller nuclei of subject one appear to be more radiosensitive. It is interesting to speculate that these cells might represent a suppressor T-cell population which is known to possess smaller nuclei and be more radiosensitive than other types of T cells. If such a thought has merit, it would be advantageous to differentiate these cells by features other than nuclear area. To test this concept, we divided all the cells on the basis of nuclear area into three subfiles (Fig. 32) and analyzed the subfiles by the discriminant analysis program. Results indicate that the cells of the three subfiles can be correctly

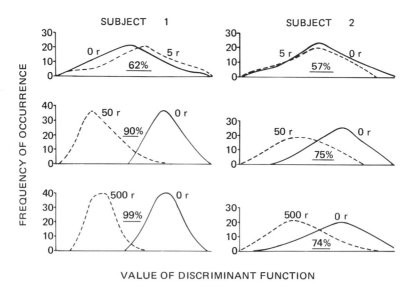

VALUE OF DISCRIMINANT FUNCTION

FIGURE 31. Comparison of nonirradiated to X-ray-irradiated lymphocytes from two subjects exposed to various doses of X-ray irradiation *in vitro*. The percentage figure indicates the discrimination success for separation between the nonirradiated and irradiated cells.

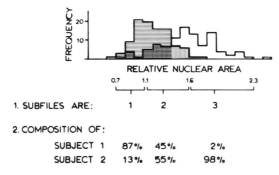

1. SUBFILES ARE: 1   2   3

2. COMPOSITION OF:

	SUBFILE 1	SUBFILE 2	SUBFILE 3
SUBJECT 1	87%	45%	2%
SUBJECT 2	13%	55%	98%

3. ANALYSIS OF SUBFILES BY DISCRM USING FEATURES OTHER THAN RELATIVE NUCLEAR AREA

ACTUAL SUBFILE	PREDICTED ASSIGNMENT MADE TO SUBFILE (%)		
	1	2	3
1	88.3	11.7	0
2	6.6	86.8	6.6
3	0	20.6	79.4

FIGURE 32. Characterization of nonirradiated Feulgen-stained lymphocytes from two subjects. Cell images of three different relative nuclear areas are differentiated into three groups by a stepwise multiple discriminant program using other features.

classified as belonging to the subfiles by four features not dependently related to nuclear area.

These studies support the belief that cell image analysis reveals important data that may be used in conjunction with biological data to further our understanding of biologic events.

D. Virus-Altered Cells: Study Four

The purpose of this study was (a) to differentiate cells infected with murine leukemia virus from normal cells, (b) to determine if virus-altered cells could be detected in virus-infected mice before other signs of the infection were evident, and (c) to correlate the results from cell image analysis with the biologic data.

Two-month-old BALB/c male mice were injected IP with 0.1 ml of Friend murine leukemia-virus suspension (2×10^3 PFU) (Olson and Bartels, 1980). At designated times after infection, the following samples were collected: blood samples from the suborbital venous plexus for total leukocyte counts and differentials; body weights and spleen weights; heart blood by cardiac puncture and splenocytes for lymphocyte preparations. At each time period (0, 2, 4, 8, 16, and 32 days postinfection) seven mice were killed. Heart blood and splenocytes from each mouse were combined to make two cell suspensions which were separated on Ficoll–Hypaque gradients (400g for 10 min) (Bozum, 1968). The lymphocytes were (a) assayed by immunofluorescence with purified rabbit anti-mouse gamma and rabbit anti-mouse-brain theta immune sera to determine percentage of T and B cells, (b) cultured *in vitro* with PHA, Con A, and LPS to assess the responsiveness to mitogenic stimulation, and (c) placed upon microscope slides, fixed, stained according to the Feulgen procedure, and scanned to determine features and decision rules important for differentiating virus-altered cells from normal cells.

Analysis of spleen-weight/body-weight ratios, total leukocyte counts, percentage of T and B cells, and changes in LPS/PHA ratios all show significant changes in virus-infected mice 10–14 days postinfection (Figs. 33 and 34).

Based upon these biologic data we scanned one hundred or more cells from each cell preparation and looked for any trendal changes in total OD, relative nuclear area, and the frequency of occurrence of OD values (Table 20, Fig. 35). The frequency of occurrence of OD values of Feulgen-stained DNA showed a pronounced change as a function of time post infection (Fig. 35). Denser-stained granules of Feulgen-positive DNA were evident in splenocytes at day 2 and by day 8 in peripheral blood cells.

Biologic and cell image data supported the concept that cells from mice 32 days postinfection represent virus-altered cells. We therefore compared the feature files of day 32 cells and day 0 (normal cells) by programs KRUS-KAL–WALLIS, AMBIGUITY, and FMERIT to list the best discriminating features. These features were used in a multiple stepwise discriminant analysis for the two data files of splenocytes to determine the degree of discrimination between normal and virus-altered cells and a ranking of the most important features.

The predicated group memberships obtained by the discriminant analysis run were

	Normal	Virus-altered
Day 0	95	5
Day 32	3	97

The ranking of the best features used to obtain the 96% correct classification is frequency of occurrence for OD values 0.31–0.40, 0.41–0.50,

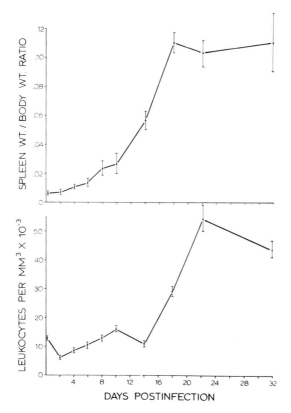

FIGURE 33. Changes in spleen-weight/body-weight ratios and numbers of leukocytes observed in BALB/c mice as a function of time postinfection with Friend murine leukemia virus.

0.61–0.70 (HIST 4, 5, and 7, respectively), total OD, average OD, radial OD profile values located 1.5–2.0 μm from the center of the nucleus and transition probabilities of OD values for the OD range of 0.21–0.40 to 0.41–0.60 (TPBR 5) and 0.21–0.40 to 0.61–0.80 (TPBR 6).

The three cells of day 32 which had features of normal cells and the five cells of day 0 which had features of virus-altered cells were identified and removed from the cell files. Day 32 (prototype for virus-altered cells) and day 0 (prototype for normal cells) were then used as training sets in a supervised learning program as described earlier. All other cells belonging to days 2, 4, 8, and 16 postinfection were classified by the algorithm to obtain their classification as normal or virus-altered cells.

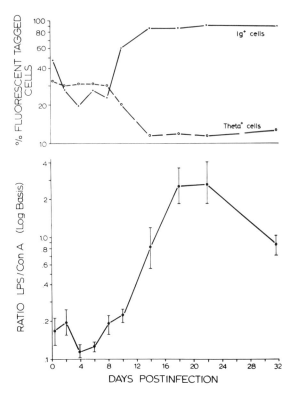

FIGURE 34. Changes in levels of immunofluorescent tagged T and B cells and ratios of LPS/ Con A mitogen activity in splenocytes obtained from BALB/c mice as a function of time post infection with Friend murine leukemia virus.

The same procedure as was used for the identification of normal and virus-altered cells of PBL was done for splenocytes, and the combined results are shown in Table 21. A trend in the detection rate of virus-altered cells is obvious with 43% of the cells of the spleen being classified as virus-altered by day 4. The appearance of virus-altered cells of the blood follows that observed in the spleen.

There appears to be a systematic and progressive change in the cells. This is reflected in the sequence in which features are selected for the differentiation of normal and virus-altered cells. This is demonstrated in Table 22. HIST 7 and average OD were the first features to be selected as the cells underwent morphologic change. As the change progressed, additional features were consistently added.

This trendal evolution of the virus-altered cell in the blood can be observed by a bivariate plot of the HIST 7 (first important feature to be

TABLE 20

Total Optical Density and Relative Nuclear Area of Peripheral Blood Lymphocytes and Splenocytes Obtained from Mice at Various Times Postinfection with Friend Leukemia Virus

Days	Total OD[a]		Relative nuclear area	
	Spleen	PBL	Spleen	PBL
0	9423	8532	287.3	324.4
2	7707	8870	181.6	262.2
4	9627	9470	300.3	267.8
8	8163	9720	135.3	216.4
16	10320	9736	187.4	160.4
32	13920	9944	274.1	187.0
$CL_{95}\%$[b]				

[a]Results are expressed as the number of 0.5 × 0.5 μm^2 OD readings per nucleus for relative nuclear area and the sum of the values of OD readings per nucleus for total OD.
[b]$CL_{95}\%$ = confidence limits expressed at 95% level. Computed on the mean square error term of the analysis of variance table.

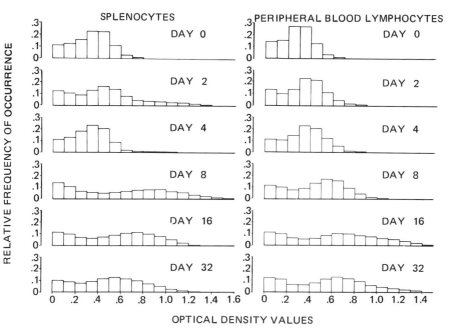

FIGURE 35. Distribution of optical density values of Feulgen-stained splenocytes and peripheral blood lymphocytes obtained from BALB/c mice as a function of time postinfection with Friend murine leukemia virus.

TABLE 21

Classification of Splenocytes and PBL as Virus-Altered Cells As a
Function of Time Postinfection with Friend Murine Leukemia Virus

Days postinfection	Splenocytes (%)		PBL (%)	
	Normal	Virus-altered	Normal	Virus-altered
0	98	0	98	0
2	90	10	91	9
4	57	43	86	14
13	10	90	24	76
16	0	100	3	97
32	2	98	0	100

selected at all time periods) vs the first discriminant function from the discriminant analysis of each virus–cell population. Figure 36 shows the normal cell population in the lower left with a positive correlation for these two features. Bayes' decision boundary marks the division in space. Cells found above this boundary should be assigned to the virus-altered groups and cells found below should be assigned to the normal group. The corresponding bivariate means, 95% confidence ellipse, and tolerance ellipses ($P = 0.50$) for all groups are within their assigned space. It is also apparent that the positive correlation between the two features is lost as a function of time postinfection.

This study clearly documents the corresponding biologic data and shows the value of image analysis in detecting viral-induced leukemic changes in cells before other signs of the leukemic process are evident (Olsen and Bartels, 1980).

TABLE 22

Chronological Occurrence of Important Features and Time when
Features Became Important in Discrimination of Virus-Altered Cells
from Normal Cells

Day 2 and 4	8	16	32
HIST 7	HIST 7	HIST 7	HIST 7
AVG OD	AVG OD	AVG OD	AVG OD
	POL-4	POL-4	POL-4
	HIST 6	HIST 6	HIST 6
	TPRB 6	TPRB 6	TPRB 6
		HIST 4	HIST 4
		HIST 5	HIST 5
			TPRB 5

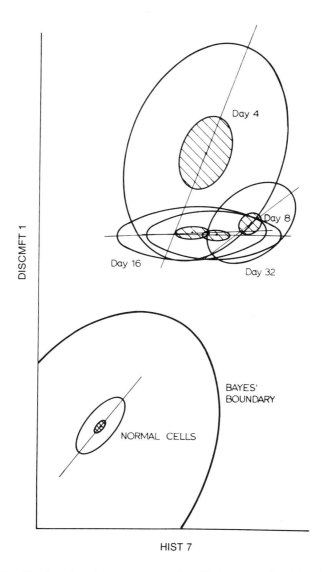

FIGURE 36.   Bivariate plot of HIST 7, DISCMFT 1 from Feulgen-stained peripheral blood lymphocytes obtained from BALB/c mice as a function of time post infection with Friend murine leukemia virus. Shaded areas represent the confidence ellipses about the bivariate mean for each cell populations. Outer ellipses represent the tolerance ellipses.

E. Detection of T and B Cells: Study Five

For the past eight years, we have analyzed lymphocytes from various lymphoid sources of mice, chicken, and man (Anderson *et al.*, 1975a,b; Bartels *et al.*, 1975, 1978b; Durie *et al.*, 1978; Olsen and Bartels, 1980; Olsen *et al.*, 1974, 1979a,b,c). Results consistently show such cell sources as PBL, TDL, and splenocytes, separated by acceptable procedures into T and B cells, can be differentiated by image analysis. The application of these methods to several of these experiments can be summarized as follows.

TDL were obtained from athymic nude mice of CBA genetic background and from CBA mice as stated in Study One (Anderson *et al.*, 1975b). Cells from CBA mice were treated with anti-IgG serum and complement to cytolyze B cells. All cells were suspended in minimum essential medium and 10% fetal calf serum during the purification and centrifugation procedures. The final cell suspensions were applied to clean microscope slides, quickly air dried, fixed with methanol and acetic acid, stained by the Feulgen procedure, and scanned. Over one hundred cells from each preparation were scanned and evaluated.

The distribution of OD values of Feulgen-positive DNA for murine T and B cells is shown in Fig. 37. Table 23 presents the relative nuclear area, total OD values, and an analysis of variance of these features for T and B cells. It is obvious that B cells possess darker-staining Feulgen granules

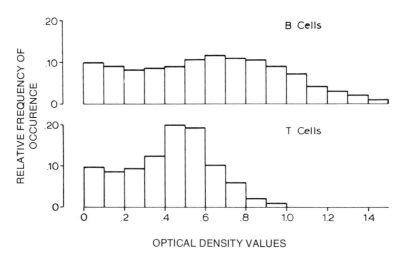

FIGURE 37. Distribution of optical density values from Feulgen-stained purified murine T and B cells.

TABLE 23
A. Total Optical Density and Relative Nuclear Area

Cell type	Total OD[a]	Relative nuclear area
T	4178	97.8
B	3980	65.0
$CL_{95}\%$[b]	±43	±1.5

B. Analysis of Variance of Mouse T and B Cells

Source of variation	Sum of squares	df	Mean squares	F value	Alpha
For total optical density ($\times 10^{-3}$)[c]					
Total	20.226816	251			
Between-cell type	5.217986	1		$_{250}^{1}86.9152$	.05
Within-cell type	15.00883	250	.06003532		
For relative nuclear area					
Total	85995.5670	251			
Between-cell type	67587.8127	1		$_{250}^{1}917.92$	.001
Within-cell type	18407.7543	250	73.63102		

[a]Results are expressed as the number of $0.5 \times 0.5 \ \mu m^2$ OD readings per nucleus for relative nuclear area and the sum of the values of OD readings per nucleus for total OD.
[b]CL_{95} % = confidence limits expressed at 95% level. Computed on the mean square error term of the analysis of variance table.
[c]Values were multiplied by 10^{-3} to preserve significant digits for calculations.

than do T cells, but T cells appear to have larger relative nuclear area and possess a larger quantity of chromophore as it develops from the Feulgen procedure (Olsen *et al.*, 1974; Bartels *et al.*, 1975).

In other experiments, we have obtained PBL from C_3H mice and have separated the cells by passage through nylon columns to obtain purified T cells. In all cases the various cell preparations were assayed for purity by immunofluorescence using highly purified monospecific rabbit anti-mouse-brain theta and rabbit anti-mouse γ immune sera.

One can demonstrate the reproducibility in the differentiation of T and B cells by comparing cells collected at different times and by different methods. For example, one can compare two populations of T cells purified by passage through nylon columns and by treatment with anti-theta plus complement with a population of B cells (Olsen *et al.*, 1979b). Application of these cell files to a stepwise discriminant analysis program using features proven capable of differentiating T and B cells causes the overall separation seen in Fig. 38. T cells and B cells depict a bimodal distribution with an approximate 13% overlap when their frequency of occurrence is plotted

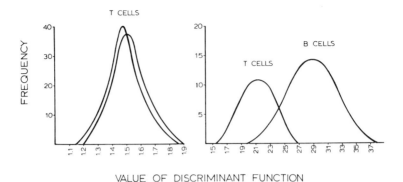

VALUE OF DISCRIMINANT FUNCTION

FIGURE 38. Frequency of the distribution of values of a discriminant function when comparing the separation of two different sets of purified murine T cells and when comparing the separation of purified T cells from B cells.

against the value of the discriminant function. There is no significant overall separation between the two T-cell files when subjected to this analysis. Visualization of the separation may be realized by a bivariate plot of the two most important features. This is shown by a bivariate plot of HIST 5 vs. average OD for the T- and B-cell files (Fig. 39). It is obvious that the two features separate the two T-cell files from B cells, but not from each other.

There appear to be characteristics which are common to T cells and to B cells, regardless of the source of the cells. This is reflected in Fig. 40 which shows the frequency of occurrence of OD values for T and B cells obtained from man, mouse, and chicken. In each case, the histograms of the B cells reveal the presence of Feulgen-positive DNA staining darker than that found in T cells.

We have subjected 550 T cells to analysis to determine if features could be found which will divide T cells into natural subsets. Two procedures were used. These included subjecting the data sets to unsupervised learning algorithms and to principal component analysis. Features were used which had previously shown high potential for the discrimination of chromatin patterns in lymphocytes. These included relative nuclear area, total and average OD, chromatin distribution as represented by radial OD value profiles, and the relative frequency of OD values in certain histogram intervals.

Table 24 shows the frequency distribution of T cells assigned to four modes by the unsupervised learning program and by a principal component analysis program. Modes are arbitrarily labeled one through four in order of decreasing proportion of the number of T cells. Differentiation by both programs results in an approximately 50, 36, 10, and 5% distribution.

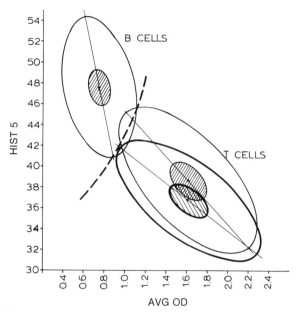

FIGURE 39. Bivariate plot of HIST 5, average optical density from Feulgen-stained purified murine T and B cells.

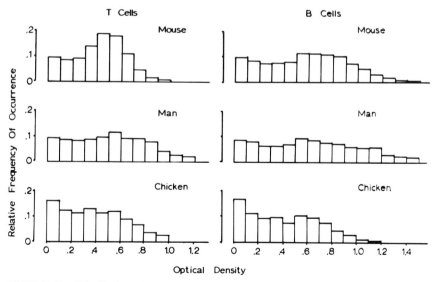

FIGURE 40. Distribution of optical density values from Feulgen-stained purified T and B cells obtained from various species.

TABLE 24

Frequency Distribution of T Cells Assigned to Four Modes by an
Unsupervised Learning Program and by a Principal Component
Analysis Program

| | % of cells to modes | | | | | |
Program	1	2	3	4	F ratio	Alpha
Unsupervised	55	38	4	2	11.49	<0.0001
Principal components	42	34	15	8		

Beale's test for significance of the classification, as made by the unsupervised learning program, shows the separation with four modes to be significant at an alpha of less than 0.0001.

The cell samples represented by the four modes were next used as "training sets" and a search was made for other features with discriminatory value. Computations of ambiguity values and a measure of detectability as explained earlier identified 24 features with good potential to discriminate different modes of T cells. These features were submitted to a stepwise linear discriminant analysis. The discriminant function employed twelve of these features and led to a Wilks' lambda of 0.2859, which indicates an excellent discrimination potential. This is confirmed by the classification matrix which is summarized in Table 25. The first six features chosen by the stepwise discriminant procedure are not highly correlated features. A list of the features and the resulting Wilks' lambda statistic important for the discrimination is as follows: HIST 5 (0.4079), nuclear area (0.3420), HIST 7 (0.3117), radial profile POL 1 (0.3041), chromatin condensation measure CND 2 (0.3009), and a texture mesh analysis feature SCS 6 (0.2991).

Visualization of some of the features of cells belonging to these four modes can be obtained by inspection of the relative frequency of occurrence of OD values of Feulgen-stained DNA. Figure 41 shows the cells

TABLE 25

Summary of Classification for Two Subgroups of T Cells As Assigned
by an Unsupervised Learning Program

| Subgroups formed by algorithms | Predicted subgroup assignment | | |
	Subgroup 1	Subgroup 2	Total
Subgroup 1	298 (94.8%)	16 (5.2%)	305
Subgroup 2	18 (8.6%)	192 (91.4%)	210

making up the larger modes contain relatively more darkly stained material and the histograms reflect a slight shift toward lower OD values. A positive correlation between relative nuclear area and total optical density, two features judged to be valuable, can be seen in the bivariate plot of Fig. 42. It must be remembered that the cells were differentiated into four modes on the basis of multiple features and therefore cannot be totally separated by only two features. This figure, however, does show good classification for

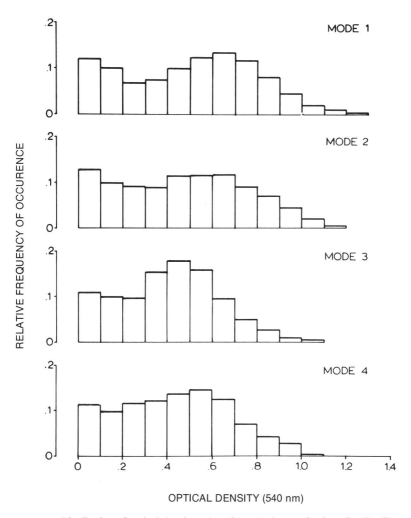

FIGURE 41. Distribution of optical density values from Feulgen-stained murine T cells separated into different modes by an unsupervised learning algorithm.

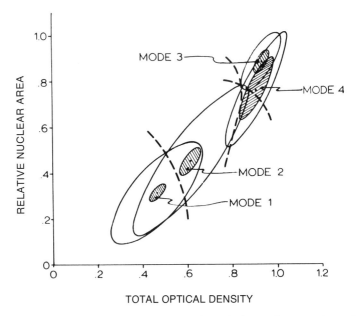

FIGURE 42. Bivariate plot of total optical density, relative nuclear area from Feulgen-stained murine T cells separated into different modes by an unsupervised learning algorithm.

cells of Mode 1 from cells of Modes 2, 3, and 4 and cells of Mode 2 as different from Mode 4.

It is apparent that image analytical techniques can be used to differentiate lymphoid cells into subpopulations of cells which agree with accepted immunologic data and methods for preparing purified cell preparations. Furthermore, it appears the programs are capable of analyzing feature data and detecting subsets of cells from purified T-cell populations. The merit of such classification must await greater knowledge about the cell cycle and biologic functions of these cells before any import can be placed upon the computer-devised classification.

REFERENCES

Anderberg, N. R., 1973, *Cluster Analysis for Applications*, Academic Press, New York.

Anderson, R. E., Olson, G. B., Howarth, J. L., Wied, G. L., and Bartels, P. H., 1975a, Computer analysis of defined populations of lymphocytes irradiated *in vitro*. II. Analysis of thymus dependent vs bone marrow derived cells, *Am. J. Pathol.* **80:**21.

Anderson, R. E., Olson, G. B., Shank, C., Howarth, J. L., Wied, G. L., and Bartels, P. H.,

1975b, Computer analysis of defined populations of lymphocytes irradiated *in vitro*. I. Evaluation of murine thoracic duct lymphocytes, *Acta Cytol.* **12**(2):126.

Anderson, R. E., Olson, G. B., Autry, J. R., Troup, M., and Bartels, P. H., 1977, Radiosensitivity of T and B lymphocytes. IV. Effect of whole body irradiation upon various lymphoid tissues and number of recirculating lymphocytes, *J. Immunol.* **118**:1191.

Bacus, J. W., 1970, An automated classification of the peripheral blood leukocytes by means of digital image processing, Ph.D. thesis, Department of Physiology, University of Illinois, Chicago.

Bartels, P. H., and Bellamy, J. C., 1970, Self-optimizing, self-learning system in pictorial pattern recognition, *Appl. Opt.* **9**:2453.

Bartels, P. H., and Subach, J. A., 1976, Automated interpretation of complex scenes, in *Digital Processing of Biomedical Imagery* (K. Preston and M. Onoe, eds.), p. 101, Academic Press, New York.

Bartels, P. H., and Wied, G. L., 1975a, Extraction and evaluation of information from digitized cell images, in *Mammalian Cells: Probes and Problems* (C. R. Richmond, D. F. Petersen, P. F. Mullaney and E. C. Anderson, eds.), p. 15, *Proceedings of the First Los Alamos Life Sciences Symposium, Los Alamos, N. M., Oct. 17–19, 1973,* Energy Research and Development Administration.

Bartels, P. H., and Wied, G. L., 1975b, High resolution prescreening systems for cervical cancer, in *Proceedings of the International Conference on Automation of Uterine Cancer,* p. 144, Chicago.

Bartels, P. H. and Wied, G. L., 1977, An image analyzing software system for cytology, in *Proceedings of the First International Computer Software and Applications Conference,* p. 282, Chicago.

Bartels, P. H., Wied, G. L., and Bahr, G. F., 1968, Cell recognition from equiprobable extinction range contours, *Acta Cytol.* **12**:202.

Bartels, P. H., Bahr, G. F., Griep, J., Rappaport, H., and Wied, G. L., 1969a, Computer analyses on lymphocytes in transformation. A methodologic study, *Acta Cytol.* **13**:557.

Bartels, P. H., Bahr, G. F., and Wied, G. L., 1969b, Cell recognition from line scan transition probability profiles, *Acta Cytol.* **13**:210.

Bartels, P. H., Bahr, G. F., Bellamy, J. C., and Wied, G. L., 1970, Self-learning program computer program for cell recognition, *Acta Cytol.* **14**:486.

Bartels, P. H., Bahr, G. F., Bibbo, M., and Wied, G. L., 1972, Objective cell image analysis, *J. Histochem. Cytochem.* **20**:239.

Bartels, P. H., Bibbo, M., Taylor, J., and Wied, G. L., 1974a, Cell recognition from the statistical dependence of gray values in digitized cell images, *Acta Cytol.* **18**:165.

Bartels, P. H., Jeter, W. S., Olson, G. B., Taylor, J., and Wied, G. L., 1974b, Evaluation of correlational information in digitized cell images, *J. Histochem. Cytochem.* **22**:69.

Bartels, P. H., Olson, G. B., Jeter, W. S., and Wied, G. L., 1974c, Evaluation of unsupervised learning algorithms in the computer analysis of lymphocytes, *Acta Cytol.* **18**:376.

Bartels, P. H., Olson, G. B., Layton, J. M., Anderson, R. E., and Wied, G. L., 1975, Computer discrimination of T and B lymphocytes, *Acta Cytol.* **19**:53.

Bartels, P. H., Bibbo, M., Richards, D., Sychra, J., and Wied, G. L., 1978a, Patient classification based on cytologic sample profiles. I. Basic measures for profile construction, *Acta Cytol.* **22**:253.

Bartels, P. H., Chen, Y. P., Durie, B. G., Olson, G. B., and Salmon, S. E., 1978b, Discrimination between human T and B lymphocytes by computer analysis of digitized data from scanning microphotometry. II. Discrimination and automated classification, *Acta Cytol.* **22**:530.

Bartels, P. H., Koss, L. G., Sychra, J. J., and Wied, G. L., 1978c, Indices of cell atypia in urinary tract cytology, *Acta Cytol.* **22**:387.

Beale, E. M. L., 1969, Euclidean cluster analysis, *Bull. Int. Stat. Inst.* **43**:92.

Boak, J. L., and Woodruff, M. F. A., 1965, A modified technique for collecting mouse thoracic duct lymph, *Nature* **205**:396.

Bozum, A., 1968, Separation of leukocytes from blood and bone marrow, *Scand. J. Clin. Lab. Invest.* **21**:(*Suppl.* 97).

Bradley, J. V., 1968, *Distribution-Free Statistical Tests,* p. 250, Prentice Hall, Englewood Cliffs, N.J.

Cooley, W. W., and Lohnes, P. R., 1962, *Multivariate Data Analysis,* p. 226, John Wiley and Sons, New York.

de Campos-Vidal, B., Schlueter, G., and Moore, G. W., 1973, Cell nucleus pattern recognition: Influence of staining, *Acta Cytol.* **17**:510.

Deitch, A. D., 1966, Cytophotometry of nucleic acids, in *Introduction to Quantitative Cytochemistry* (G. L. Wied, ed.), p. 327, Academic Press, New York.

Dixon, W. J., 1967, *BMD Biomedical Computer Programs,* p. 185, University of California Press, Berkeley.

Duda, O., and Hart, P. E., 1973, *Pattern Classification and Scene Analysis,* p. 250, John Wiley and Sons, New York.

Durie, B. G., Vaught, M. L., Chen, Y. P., Olson, G. B., Salmon, S. E., and Bartels, P. H., 1978, Discrimination between human T and B lymphocytes, and monocytes by computer analysis of digitized data from scanning microphotometry. I. Chromatin distribution patterns, *Blood* **51**:579.

Freeman, H., 1961, On the encoding of arbitrary geometric configurations, *IEEE Trans. Electron. Comput.* **10**:260.

Fukunaga, K., 1972, *Introduction to Statistical Pattern Recognition,* p. 90, Academic Press, New York.

Genchi, H., and Mori, K., 1965, Evaluation and feature extraction on automated pattern recognition system, *Denki Tsuchin Gakkai Zasshi Part 1* (in Japanese), quoted in Tanaka, N., Ideda, H., Ueno, T., Watanabe, S., Imasato, Y., and Kashida, I., 1976, Fundamental study of an automated cytoscreening system utilizing the pattern recognition system. I. Feature evaluation in the pattern recognition system, in *The Automation of Uterine Cancer Cytology* (G. L. Wied, G. F. Bahr, and P. H. Bartels, eds.), pp. 223–227, Tutorials of Cytology, Chicago.

Haralick, R. M., Shanmugam, K., and Dinstein, I., 1973, Textural features for image classification, *IEEE Trans. Syst. Man Cybern.* **3**:610.

Harbers, E., and Sandritter, W., 1968, Gesteigerte Heterochromatisierung als pathogenetisches Prinzip. *Dtsch. Med. Wochenschr.* **93**:269.

Harbers, E., Lederer, B., Sandritter, W., and Spaar, U., 1968, Untersuchungen and Nukleohistonen. IV. Heterochromatisierung in der Rattenleber Waehrend für Carcinogenese, *Virchows Arch. B.* **1**:98.

Hartigan, J. A., 1975, *Clustering Algorithms,* p. 434, Academic Press, New York.

Ingram, M., Norgren, P. E., and Preston, K., 1968, Automatic differentiation of white blood cells, in *Image Processing in Biologic Science* (D. M. Ramsey, ed.), p. 97, University of California Press, Berkeley.

Julesz, B., 1962, Visual pattern discrimination, *IRE Trans. Inf. Theory* **8**:84.

Julesz, B., 1975, Experiments in the visual perception of texture, *Sci. Am.* **232**:34.

Julesz, B., Gilbert, E. N., Shepp, L. A., and Frisch, H. L., 1973, Inability of humans to discriminate between visual textures that agree in second order statistics—revisited, *Perception* **2**:391.

Kiefer, J. G., Kiefer, R., and Sandritter, W. W., 1971, Die Dichterverteilung des Chromatins innerhalb des Zellkerns, *Verh. Dtsch. Ges. Pathol.* **55**:621.

Kiefer, R., Kiefer, J. G., Salm, R., Rossner, R., and Sandritter, W., 1973, A method for the quantitative evaluation of eu- and heterochromatin in interphase nuclei using cytophotometry and pattern analysis, *Beitr. Pathol. Anat.* **150**:163.

Kiefer, J. G., Kiefer, R., Moore, G. W., Salm, R., and Sandritter, W., 1974, Nuclear images of cells in different functional states, *J. Histochem. Cytochem.* **22**:569.

Kiehn, T. E., 1972, Computer analysis of transforming lymphocytes, Ph.D. thesis, Department of Microbiology, University of Arizona, Tucson.

Klecka, W. R., Nie, N. H., and Hull, C. H., 1975, SPSS *Statistical Package for the Social Sciences,* McGraw-Hill, New York.

Koss, L. G., Bartels, P. H., Bibbo, M., Freed, S. Z., Taylor, J., and Wied, G. L., 1975, Computer discrimination between benign and malignant urothelial cells, *Acta Cytol.* **19**:378.

Koss, L. G., Bartels, P. H., Bibbo, M., Freed, S. Z., Sychra, J. J., Taylor, J., and Wied, G. L., 1977a, Computer analysis of atypical urothelial cells. I. Classification by supervised learning algorithms, *Acta Cytol.* **21**:247.

Koss, L. G., Bartels, P. H., Sychra, J. J., and Wied, G. L., 1977b, Computer analysis of atypical urothelial cells. II. Classification by unsupervised learning algorithms, *Acta Cytol.* **21**:261.

Koss, L. G., Bartels, P. H., Sychra, J. J., and Wied, G. L., 1978a, Computer discriminant analysis of atypical urothelial cells, *Acta Cytol.* **22**:382.

Koss, L. G., Bartels, P. H., Sychra, J. J., and Wied, G. L., 1978b, Diagnostic cytologic sample profiles in patients with bladder cancer using TICAS system, *Acto Cytol.* **22**:392.

Kulkarni, A. V., and Kanal, L., 1976, An optimization approach to hierarchial classifier design. Proceedings of the Third International Joint Conference on Pattern Recognition. *IEEE Trans. Comput.* **76**:459 (C 1140–3C).

Landeweerd, G. H., and Gelsema, E. S., 1978, The use of nuclear texture parameters in the automatic analysis of leukocytes, *Pattern Recognition* **10**:57.

McClellan, R. P., 1971. Optimization and stochastic approximation techniques applied to unsupervised learning. Ph.D. thesis, Department of Electrical Engineering, University of Arizona, Tucson.

McKee, P. H. 1975. Computer analyses of lymphocyte alterations induced by immunosuppressive chemical agents. Ph.D. thesis, Department of Microbiology, University of Arizona, Tucson.

Olson, G. B., and Bartels, P. H., 1980, Differentiation of splenocytes and peripheral blood lymphocytes from mice infected with Friend leukemia virus, *Pattern Recognition* (in press).

Olson, G. B., Anderson, R. E., and Bartels, P. H., 1974, Differentiation of murine thoracic duct lymphocytes into T and B subpopulations by computer cell scanning techniques, *Cell. Immunol.* **13**:347.

Olson, G. B., Anderson, R. E., and Bartels, P. H., 1979a, Computer analysis of defined populations of lymphocytes irradiated *in vitro*. III. Evaluation of human T and B cells of peripheral blood origin, *Hum. Pathol.* **10**:179.

Olson, G. B., Anderson, R. E., and Bartels, P. H., 1979b, Characterization of murine T and B cells by computerized microphotometric analysis, *Cell Biophysics* **1**:229.

Olson, G. B., Bartels, P. H., and Anderson, R. E., 1979c, Subclassification of murine T cells by computerized microphotometric analysis, *Cell Biophysics* **1**:243.

Pressman, N. J., 1976a, Optical texture analysis for automatic cytology and histology: A Markovian approach, Ph.D. thesis, Lawrence Livermore Laboratory, University of California, Los Angeles.

Pressman, N. J., 1976b, Markovian analysis of cervical cell images, *J. Histochem. Cytochem.* **24**:138.

Preston, K. 1961, The CELLSCAN system: A leukocyte pattern analyzer, p. 173, *Proceedings of the Western Joint Computer Conference*.

Preston, K., Jr., 1962, Machine techniques for automatic leukocyte pattern analysis, *Ann. N.Y. Acad. Sci.* **97**:482.

Preston, K., 1976, Digital image analysis in cytology, in *Digital Image Analysis* (Azriel Rosenfeld, ed.), Springer Verlag, New York.

Prewitt, J. M. S., 1972, Parametric and nonparametric recognition by computer: An application to leukocyte image processing, *Adv. Comput.* **12**:285.

Prewitt, J. M. S., and Mendelsohn, M. L., 1966, The analysis of cell images, *Ann. N.Y. Acad. Sci.* **128**:1035.

Raff, M. D., Sternberg, M., and Taylor, R. B., 1970, Immunoglobulin determinants on surface of mouse lymphoid cells, *Nature* **225**:553.

Reale, F., Bartels, P. H., Bibbo, M. Chen, M., Schreiber, H., and Wied, G. L., 1979, Differentiation by TICAS analysis of cell populations of tracheal aspirates from hamsters with squamous carcinoma, *Amer. J. Clin. Pathol.* **72**:52.

Reinhardt, E., Erhardt, R., Schwarzmann, P., Bloss, W., and Ott, R., 1979, Structure analysis and classification of cervical cells using a processing system based on TV, *Anal. Quant. Cytol.* **1**:143.

Richmond, C. R., Petersen, D. F., Mullaney, P. F., and Anderson, E. C. (eds.), 1975, *Mammalian Cells: Probes and Problems. Proceedings of the First Los Alamos Life Sciences Symposium, Los Alamos, N.M., Oct. 17–19, 1973*, Energy Research and Development Administration.

Rosenfeld, A., and Troy, E. B., 1970, Visual texture analysis, *Computer Science Center Technical Report* 70/116, University of Maryland, College Park, Maryland.

Rowinski, J., Pienkowski, M., and Abramszuk, J., 1972, Area representation of optical density of chromatin in resting and stimulated lymphocytes as measured by means of Quantimet, *Histochemie* **32**:75.

Sandritter, W., and Kiefer, G., 1970, Objectivization of chromatin patterns using the fast-scanning stage of the UMSP1, in *Automated Cell Identification and Cell Sorting* (G. L. Wied and G. F. Bahr, eds.), p. 177, Academic Press, New York.

Sandritter, W., Kiefer, G., Schlüter, G., and Moore, W., 1967, Eine cytophotometrische Methode zur Objektivierung der Morphologie von Zellkernen, *Histochemie* **10**:341.

Serra, J., 1974, Theoretical bases of the Leitz Tecture analyzing system, Scientific and Technical Information, Leitz, Wetzlar (Suppl.) **4**:125.

Sherwood, E., Bartels, P. H., and Wied, G. L., 1976, Feature selection in cell image analysis use of the ROC curve, *Acta Cytol.* **20**:255.

Simon, H., Kunze, K. D., Voss, K., and Herrmann, W. R., 1975, *Automatische Boldverarbeitung in Medizin und Biologie*, p. 155, Theodor Steinkopff Verlag, Dresden.

Stobo, J. D. and Paul, W. E., 1973, Functional heterogeneity of murine lymphoid cells. III. Differential responsiveness of T cells to phytohemagglutinin and concanvalin A as a probe for T cell subsets, *J. Immunol.* **110**:362.

Sychra, J. J., Bartels, P. H., Taylor, J., Bibbo, M., and Wied, G. L., 1976, Cytoplasmic and nuclear shape analysis for computerized cell recognition, *Acta Cytol.* **20**:68.

Sychra, J., Bartels, P. H., Bibbo, M., Taylor, J., and Wied, G. L., 1977, Computer recognition of abnormal ectocervical cells. Comparison of efficacy of contour and textural features, *Acta Cytol.* **21**:765.

Taylor, J., Bartels, P. H. Bibbo, M., Bahr, G. F., and Wied, G. L., 1974, Implementation of a hierarchical cell classification procedure, *Acta Cytol.* **18**:515.

Taylor, J., Bartels, P. H., Bibbo, M., and Wied, G. L., 1978a, Automated hierarchic decision structures for multiple cell classification by TICAS, *Acta Cytol.* **22**:261.

Taylor, J., Puls, J., Sychra, J., Bartels, P. H., Bibbo, M., and Wied, G. L., 1978b, A system for scanning biological cells in three colors, *Acta Cytol.* **22**:29.

Vastola, E. F., Hertzberg, R., Neurath, P., and Brenner, J., 1974, A description by computer of texture in Wright stained leukocytes, *Acta Cytol.* **18**:231.

Wasmund, H., 1976, Computergesteuertes Scanning Mikroskop fuer die Analyse von Einzelzellen, *Leitz-Mitt. Wiss. Tech.* **6**:217.

Wied, G. L., Bartels, P. H., Bahr, G. F., and Oldfield, D. G., 1968, Taxonomic intracellular analytic system (TICAS) for cell identification, *Acta Cytol.* **12**:177.

Wied, G. L., Bahr, G. F., and Bartels, P. H., 1970a, Automatic analysis of cell images by TICAS, in *Automated Cell Identification and Cell Sorting* (G. L. Wied and G. F. Bahr, eds.), p. 195, Academic Press, New York.

Wied, G. L., Bibbo, M., Bahr, G. F., and Bartels, P. H., 1970b, Computerized recognition of uterine glandular cells. III. Assessment of the efficacy of 1 μ vs $\frac{1}{2}$ μ measuring spot size, *Acta Cytol.* **14**:136.

Wied, G. L., Bibbo, M., Bahr, G. F., and Bartels, P. H., 1970c, Computerized microdissection of cellular images, *Acta Cytol.* **14**:418.

Wied, G. L., Bahr, G. F., and Bartels, P. H. (eds.) 1976, *The Automation of Uterine Cancer Cytology,* Tutorials of Cytology, Chicago.

Wied, G. L., Bartels, P. H., Bibbo, M., Chen, M., Reale, F. R., Schreiber, H., and Sychra, J. J., 1979, Discriminant analysis on cells from developing squamous cancer of the respiratory tract, *Cell Biophysics* **1**:39.

Young, I. T., 1969, Automated leukocyte recognition, Ph.D. thesis, Massachusetts Institute of Technology, Cambridge, Massachusetts.

Young, I. T., Walker, J. E., and Bowie, J. E., 1974, An analysis technique for biological shape. I, *Inf. Control* **25**:357.

2

Principles of Continuous Flow Cell Separation in a Circumferential Flow Disposable Channel

JEANE P. HESTER, ROBERT M. KELLOGG, ALFRED
MULZET, KENNETH B. McCREDIE, AND EMIL J
FREIREICH

I. INTRODUCTION

Continuous flow centrifugation (CFC) is used to centrifuge large volumes of blood and concentrate cellular or acellular subfractions for extraction. The efficient separation of most blood components requires a system that permits removal of selected elements while returning most of the remaining fractions to the donor/patient. When used in the biological sciences, these systems must be closed and sterile. In 1965, Freireich *et al.* reported the first use of a closed, sterile, continuous flow centrifuge in man to perform leukocyte extraction. Application growth is based on the fact that these systems allow access to a donor/patient's entire blood volume for processing and manipulation. A nonexhaustive list of CFC applications is contained in Table 1.

The initial role of CFC was collection of granulocytes from the blood

JEANE P. HESTER, KENNETH B. McCREDIE, AND EMIL J FREI-
REICH • Department of Developmental Therapeutics, M. D. Anderson Hospital and
Tumor Institute, The University of Texas System Cancer Center, Houston, Texas
77030.   ROBERT M. KELLOGG AND ALFRED MULZET • Biomedical Systems
Division, IBM Corporation, Endicott, New York 13760. The research for this chapter was
supported in part by Grants CA05831 and CA19806 from the National Institutes of Health,
Bethesda, Maryland 20014.

TABLE 1
Applications of CFC

1. Collection
   Granulocytes, mononuclear cells, platelets—transfusion, immune modulation
   Stem cells—bone marrow reconstitution
2. Depletion
   Leukemic leukocytosis—acute or chronic
   Thromobocytosis
3. Exchange
   Plasma
   Red cells

of normal donors for replacement transfusions to neutropenic patients (<1000 PMN/μl) who had established infections unresponsive to appropriate antibiotic regimens (Graw *et al.*, 1972) and this continues to be a major application of this system. Mononuclear cell collection has been carried out for transfusions for mucopolysaccharide disorders (DiFerante *et al.*, 1973), stem cell collection, and storage for bone marrow reconstitution (McCredie and Freireich, 1971; Sarpel *et al.*, 1979) and immunological modulation (Curtis *et al.*, 1969, 1970; Hersh *et al.*, 1979). Plasma exchange for a large number of autoimmune and other disorders and red cell exchange in patients with hemoglobinopathies are rapidly enlarging areas of CFC application.

Experience gained over the years disclosed limitations of the original CFC system which related primarily to the nondisposable blood path and system performance which was strongly affected by the operator skill and attention. A second generation CFC system has been designed to remedy these limitations and to identify appropriate procedural parameters for specific application of CFC to cellular collection, depletion, or exchange.

II. DESIGN CONCEPTS

CFC systems to perform leukapheresis have been described in detail (Jones, 1968; Judson *et al.*, 1968). The new disposable single-stage channel differs in two important ways from current CFC devices.

1. Blood flow during separation is circumferential in the disposable system, i.e., the flow is in a circle around the axis of rotation.
2. The red cell buffy coat–plasma interface position within the single-stage channel is stabilized by the design of the channel so that buffy coat collection relates to channel design and only minimal operator attention is required.

   The central element in all CFC devices is the centrifuge in which separation takes place. A brief review of separation in the current axial flow devices is pertinent to the design of the circumferential flow disposable channel. Blood flow during separation in axial flow systems (polycarbonate bowl) is parallel to the axis of rotation. The RBC–plasma interface position and buffy coat (leukocyte–platelet) collection are under the direct control of the operator who must vary the relative extraction flow rates of packed RBC and plasma to obtain the desired component. In this system, whole blood separates in the annular separation channel as the blood flows axially from the bottom to the collection area at the top of the bowl where the separated components are seen beneath a transparent cover. The ability of the centrifuge to separate whole blood in the axial flow system can be explained by introducing the concept of a packing factor defined as

$$P_f = \frac{sGt}{d} \tag{1}$$

where G = centrifugal acceleration, t = time of exposure to G, d = distance through which separation takes place, and s = sedimentation parameter of material being separated.

   Substitution of the physical parameters of the bowl (Fig. 1) into equation (1) gives

$$P_f = \frac{s\,\Omega^2 r^2 l}{Q} \tag{2}$$

where Q = whole blood flow rate, Ω = angular velocity, r = radial location of separation channel, and l = axial length of the separation channel.

   Note that equation (2) does not depend on channel width. Jones (1968) showed this lack of dependency experimentally. Equation (2) can be used to compare the separation characteristics of axial flow centrifuges of differing geometry.

   Axial flow centrifuges, however, are not adaptable to inexpensive or disposable fabrication techniques. It was felt, however, that relatively inexpensive assemblies could be fabricated if whole blood separation were to take place in circular channels with flow circumferential to the axis of rotation. Such channels could then be formed from laminated plastic film or extruded stock.

   To determine what the proportions of such a system would be, analysis of a laminated circumferential separation channel (Fig. 2) was carried out to determine the packing factor

$$P_f = \frac{s\,\Omega^2 r^2 A}{dQ} \tag{3}$$

where A = channel cross-sectional area and d = radial width.

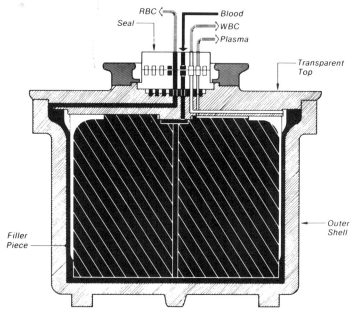

FIGURE 1.   The axial flow centrifuge bowl (cross section).

Equating equations (2) and (3) gives

$$\Omega_a^2 \, r_a^2 l_a = \frac{\Omega_c^2 r_c^2 A_c}{dc} \tag{4}$$

where subscripts a and c refer to the axial and circumferential systems respectively.

Equation (4) assumes that the sedimentation constant (s) and flow rates of (Q) the two systems are equal. By using equation (4), it is possible to proportion a laminated circumferential flow system with separation characteristics similar to the axial flow centrifuge. Such a system was fabricated. This channel, when expanded in the centrifuge bowl, had the following characteristics:

$$A = 0.45 \text{ cm}^2$$
$$d = 1.1 \text{ cm}$$
$$r_c = 16.3 \text{cm}$$

For these values, equation (4) gives angular speeds for the laminated circumferential flow system 1.8 times that of the axial flow system for comparable separation. The centrifugal acceleration in the circumferential system is approximately 8.5 times that of the axial flow system.

The efficiency of leukocyte separation, in particular granulocyte separation, is sensitive to the centrifugal acceleration at which separation takes

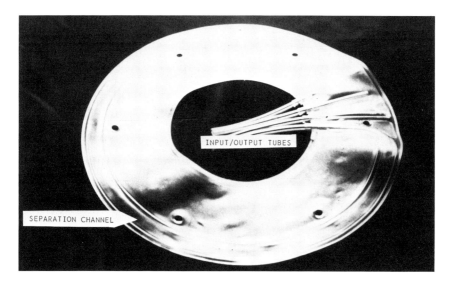

FIGURE 2. Laminated circumferential separation channel.

place. This can be seen in Fig. 3 which gives the total number of cells collected per liter of whole blood processed as a function of centrifuge rpm for the laminated circumferential system. These measurements were made at constant packing factors so that for this fixed geometry decreasing the centrifuge speed implied a corresponding decrease in flow rates. Acceptable collection rates were obtained at 560 rpm. However, the system's whole blood flow rate was unacceptably low at 6 ml/min. Since system flow rates of at least 50 ml/min are required to achieve acceptable leukocyte yield and total procedure time, the packing factor of the circumferential system was increased approximately eight times by using an extruded channel of rectangular cross-section 3.0 × 10.6 cm. The channel length was essentially the same, being dictated by the desire to keep the channel volume less than 200 ml and to limit extracorporeal donor blood volume.

The channel area (A), length (l), and distance (d) through which sedimentation takes place are geometrical properties of the system and are fixed. Sedimentation (S) is a donor biological variable and is not directly controllable. Thus, the degree of separation in the extruded single-stage channel can be characterized by the ratio of separation acceleration G to flow rate Q through the channel. If this ratio is held constant, similar separation should be obtained at different G and Q. The combination of centrifuge speed (rpm) and flow rates (ml/min) that maintain that constant ratio indicated that 580/40, 650/50, 720/60 and 820/80 should provide comparable yields of approximately 3.0×10^9 cells/liter of blood processed.

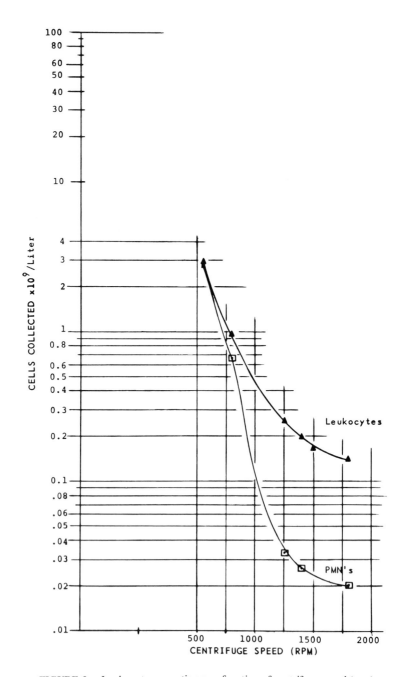

FIGURE 3. Leukocyte separation as a function of centrifuge speed (rpm).

III. CHANNEL DESCRIPTION

The single-stage channel consists of an extruded, semirigid rectangular polyvinyl chloride plastic tube which is attached to the input and collection chamber to form a closed loop as shown in Fig. 4. Four tubes from the face seal provide passages for whole blood into the channel and extraction of packed red blood cells (RBC) buffy coat and plasma or a mixture of RBC and plasma. There is no direct communication between the input port and the collection chamber. Three exit ports have different radial positions within the collection chamber. The buffy coat and the interface positioning port (IFPP) are radially positioned to lie on the center line of the channel. They are separated from each other by a barrier that extends from the top to the bottom of the chamber. Plasma can pass around the barrier along the inner wall and RBC flow around the barrier along the outer wall of the chamber. Downstream from the barrier, RBC and plasma are recombined and extracted by the IFPP.

IV. CHANNEL OPERATION

The separation channel is mounted in the centrifuge with the axis of rotation in the center of the loop. Extracorporeal anticoagulation of whole blood is achieved by a 1:13 dilution of ACD concentrate to whole blood in the input line. Anticoagulated whole blood is drawn into the channel by extracting priming saline through the IFPP. As the system fills with blood, separation occurs and plasma replaces saline in the IFPP. After approximately 250 ml of blood have been processed, RBC–plasma appears in the IFPP. Semiautomatic positioning of the RBC–plasma interface occurs as follows: The downstream stabilized interface is related to the physical position of the IFPP. The location of this interface, in turn, forces the interface on the upstream side of the barrier to take the same radial location. This is, in principle, the same as a mercury U-tube manometer in which the height of the mercury column is equal in both arms of the tube if the pressure exerted against both mercury columns is equal. The pressure exerted by plasma on the interface is uniform, but as processing continues, a dense layer of packed RBC forms on the outside wall of the collect well. The upstream interface moves radially inward to maintain uniform pressure along the outside wall. The amount of radial offset between the upstream and downstream interface location can be controlled by the extraction rate of packed RBC through the RBC port. A leukocyte (WBC)–platelet buffy coat forms on the upstream side of the barrier and both components are extracted through the WBC collect port which lies adjacent to the barrier. Thus, WBC collection relates to channel design and not to visualization of

Single Stage

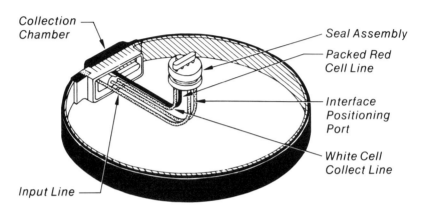

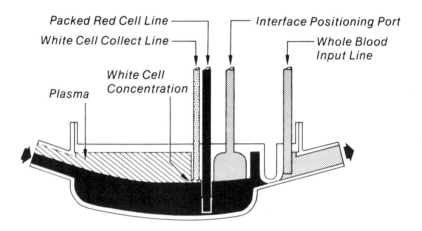

FIGURE 4.   Circumferential disposable flow channel.

TABLE 2
Operating Parameters

Separation channel	Speed (rpm)	Flow rates (ml/min)	Blood processed (liters)	Time (min)
Circumferential				
Mean	720	60	8.8	142
Range	580–820	40–80	4.4–10	78–200
Axial				
Mean	750	50	10.0	180
Range		50–56		100–200

TABLE 3
Total Cellular Yields of Single-Stage
Disposable Channel

Cell type	Mean yield	Range
WBC $\times$ 10^9	33.0 ± 11.6	13.7–63.6
PMN $\times$ 10^9	26.7 ± 10.2	9.0–55.4
Lymph $\times$ 10^9	4.4 ± 2.3	0.9–13.7
Mono $\times$ 10^9	2.0 ± 2.0	0.0–8.8
Plate $\times$ 10^{11}	1.1 ± 0.6	0.2–3.3
RBC $\times$ 10^{11}	1.1 ± 0.5	0.1–2.1

a buffy coat as found in axial flow devices. Collection begins when suffi-cient packing of RBC has occurred (500–1000 ml processed) to introduce RBC into the WBC collect line. Controlling the extraction rate of the RBC controls the cellular makeup of the buffy coat collection.

A. Results

Statistical analysis was carried out on 130 granulocyte collection pro-cedures and compared to 980 procedures in the axial flow systems. Oper-ating parameters, mean procedure time, and volume of whole blood anti-coagulant processed are shown in Table 2. Total cellular yields are shown in Table 3.

V. CHANNEL PERFORMANCE

A. Granulocyte Collection

The mean cell yield for all procedures in the circumferential system was 33.0 $\times$ 10^9 ± 11.6 WBC (range 13.7 –63.6), of which 26.7 $\times$ 10^9 ± 10.2

were granulocytes and the remainder were mononuclear cells. Mean WBC yield for the axial flow system was 18.5 $\times$ 10^9 $\pm$ 13.5 WBC (range 1.0–45.0), with 13.8 $\times$ 10^9 $\pm$ 11 PMN. The circumferential disposable channel showed a 54% increase in yield with a 21% reduction in procedure time.

Granulocyte harvesting in the single-stage disposable channel depends strongly on two additional factors whose importance was first demonstrated in the axial flow CFC by McCredie *et al.* (1974) and Mischler *et al.* (1974). These are the height of the donor precount and the use of a macromolecular sedimenting agent, usually hydroxyethyl starch, in the input line during processing.

The height of the donor precount is a biological variable that can be manipulated to some extent. Donor premedication with corticosteroids or other agents, etiocholanolone, induces a variable leukocytosis with a shift in the peripheral blood differential toward granulocytosis. This variable is strongly correlated with the final granulocyte yield (p = 0.0001) (Hester *et al.*, 1979). These relationships were similar for the circumferential and axial flow system as shown in Table 4 but superior yields can be noted for the disposable channel at each level of donor peripheral count.

Four centrifuge speeds (rpm) and processing flow rates (ml/min) were determined relative to the separation characteristics already described. These were 580/40, 650/50, 720/60, and 820/80. Donor selection for each combination was based on donor blood volume measurements. ACD anticoagulant binds calcium and a reduction in ionized calcium occurs that is related to the infusion rate of the anticoagulant and blood volume of the donor. Donors with blood volumes $\geq$ 5.0 liters could be processed at 820/80 ml/min which resulted in a significant reduction in procedure time. While the equations predicted comparable yields, experiments documented that yields did increase at centrifuge speeds of 820 rpm (p = .003), but there was some reduction in the granulocyte fraction in the final product.

At low G forces, with sedimenting agents, granulocytes may be effectively collected. Because of size and density, most platelets are left free in

TABLE 4
Relationship of Donor Leukocyte Count Preleukopheresis to Total Yield

Donor precount (WBC $\times$ $10^3/\mu l$)	Mean yield $\times 10^9$ cells	
	Circumferential flow, disposable channel	Axial flow, reusable bowl
6–8	22	11
8–10	26	14
10–12	33	17
12–14	40	20
14–16	45	27

TABLE 5
Mononuclear Cell Collection Single-Stage Circumferential System

Centrifuge speed (rpm)	Blood processed (liters)	Cellular yield mononuclear platelet	
		$\times 10^9$	$\times 10^{11}$
580–820	8.8	9. 4 ± 4	1.6 ± .5
900–1100	2.0–4.0	2.63 ± 2	2.5 ± 1.0
900–1100	4.0–6.0	5.82 ± 2	3.9 ± 2.0

the plasma to be returned to the donor as evidenced by a low mean platelet yield of 1.1×10^{11} cells in granulocyte procedures.

B. Mononuclear Cell Collection

When G forces are increased and sedimenting agents with ACD concentrate are replaced with ACD-A anticoagulant, granulocytes are replaced by mononuclear cells so that the leukocyte-rich buffy coat contains about 90% lymphocytes and monocytes. A larger number of platelets are brought down out of the plasma to the interface to be extracted with the buffy coat.

Mononuclear cell yields and platelet yields from procedures performed at low centrifuge speeds (580–820 rpm) and high centrifuge speeds (900–1100 rpm) are compared in Table 5. A positive relationship between mononuclear cell yield and the amount of blood processed is demonstrated while the increase in platelet yield correlates with the increase in rpm. Statistical analysis indicates a statistically significant correlation between donor lymphocyte count ($r = 0.350$, $p = 0.0008$) and final yield. The proportion of monocytes collected did not correlate with donor peripheral blood monocyte concentration and these cells may be mobilized during the procedure.

C. Plasma Exchange

Plasma exchange offers a modality for rapid reduction in abnormal substances in the intravascular system. Its therapeutic effectiveness is being investigated in a large number of medical diseases which include malignant paraproteinemias and autoimmune disorders.

In the circumferential flow system, plasma exchange is carried out at 1600 rpm. At these G forces, most platelets are removed from the plasma, combined with the buffy coat, extracted with packed RBC through the RBC port and returned to the patient. This is accomplished by keeping the RBC–plasma interface 3–5 mm from the IFPP through which the platelet-poor plasma is being extracted. Replacement solutions (fresh frozen plasma, protein solutions, saline, etc.) are delivered through the WBC pump at rates that equal plasma extraction so that volume balance is maintained. Flow rates, and thus procedure time, relate to anticoagulant infusion rates and patient blood volume and are selected to avoid inappropriate calcium depletion in the patient. Analysis of exchange procedures performed in this channel indicated that for a mean procedure time of 62 min, 4.3 liters of whole blood were processed with extraction and exchange of 2.65 liters of plasma. The mean total cellular loss in the extracted plasma was 0.9×10^9 leukocytes and 1.4×10^{11} platelets.

Platelet and leukocyte losses are thereby minimized. This has important applications for patients who are leukopenic and thrombocytopenic from immunosuppressive agents delivered as primary treatment for the underlying disease process.

VI. SUMMARY

The circumferential flow, single-stage, disposable channel has broad applications for CFC procedures and improved performance over existing axial flow devices. This second-generation CFC pathway has expanded scientific understanding of the characteristics of whole blood separation in response to centrifugal forces. Procedural parameters have been identified that maximize its usefulness in cellular collection or exchange. The relationship of donor–patient biological variability to the technological concepts of the system is characterized and mathematical expression of these relationships offers guidelines for optimal performance of the system.

REFERENCES

Curtis, J. E., Hersh, E. M., and Freireich, E. J., 1970, Antigen specific immunity in recipients of leukocyte transfusions from immune donors, *Cancer Res.* 30:2921–2929.

Curtis, J. E., Hersh, E. M., and Freireich, E. J., 1969, Transfer of immunity with leukocytes in man, in *International Symposium of the Centre National de la Récherche Scientifique, White Cell Transfusion, Paris,* pp. 167–185, Editions du Centre National de la Récherche Scientifique, Paris.

DiFerante, N., Nicholas, B., Knudson, A., McCredie, K. B., Singh, J., and Donnelly, P. V., 1973, Mucopolysaccharide storage diseases. Corrective activity of normal human serum and lymphocyte extracts, *Birth Defects* 9:31–40.

Freireich, E. J., Judson, G., and Levin, R. H., 1965, Separation and collection of leukocytes, *Cancer Res.* 25:1516–1520.

Graw, R. G., Herzig, G., Perry, S., and Henderson, E., 1972, Normal granulocyte transfusion therapy: Treatment of septicemia due to gram negative sepsis, *N. Engl. J. Med.* 287:367.

Hersh, E. M., Murphy, S., and Toki, H., 1979, Immunological deficiency in hairy cell leukemia and its correction by leukocyte transfusions, *Proc. Am. Assoc. Cancer Res./Am. Soc. Clin. Oncol.* **20**:382.

Hester, J. P., Kellogg, R. M., Mulzet, A. P., Kruger, V. R., McCredie, K. B., and Freireich, E. J., 1979, Principles of blood separation and component extraction in a disposable continuous-flow single-stage channel, *Blood* **54**(1):254–268.

Jones, A., 1968, Continuous flow blood cell separation, *Transfusion* **8**:94–103.

Judson, G., Jones, A., and Kellogg, R., 1968, Closed continuous flow centrifuge, *Nature* **217**:816–818.

McCredie, K. B., and Freireich, E. J., 1971, Cells capable of colony formation in the peripheral blood of man, *Science* **171**:290–294.

McCredie, K. B., Freireich, E. J., Hester, J. P., and Vallejos, C., 1974, Increased granulocyte collection with the blood cell separator and the addition of etiocholanolone and hydroxyethyl starch, *Transfusion* **14**:357–364.

Mischler, J. M., Higby, D. J., Rhomberg, W., Cohen, E., Nicora, R. W., and Holland, J. F., 1974, Hydroxyethyl starch and dexamethasone as an adjunct to leukocyte separation with the IBM blood cell separator, *Transfusion* **14**:352–357.

Sarpel, S. C., Zander, A. R., Harvath, L., and Epstein, R. B., 1979, The collection, preservation and function of peripheral blood hematopoietic cells in dogs, *Exp. Hematol. (Copenhagen)* **2**:113–120.

3

Magnetic Microspheres in Cell Separation

PAUL L. KRONICK

I. BACKGROUND

A. Physics of Magnetophoresis

1. Some Definitions

The term magnetization refers to the appearance of a magnetic dipole of magnitude m in a body, either spontaneously or when it is placed in a magnetic field of magnitude H. The magnetization of a material M is a point variable which depends on the applied magnetic field H and the chemical composition. It is defined as

$$M = m/V \tag{1}$$

where V is the volume of the body. Because in most materials M is zero when $H = 0$ and increases monotonically with H, a material parameter, the magnetic susceptibility χ is defined as

$$\chi = M/H \tag{2}$$

Most organic materials have small negative values of χ and so are diamagnetic. Paramagnetic materials have small positive values of χ such as hematite, Fe_2O_3, ($\chi = 4.54 \times 10^{-9}$ H/m). Ferromagnetic materials have much

---

PAUL L. KRONICK • Department of Physical and Life Sciences, Franklin Research Center, Philadelphia, Pennsylvania 19103.

larger values; χ for iron exceeds 10^{-2} H/m. Both paramagnetic and ferro-magnetic materials can be used for cell separation.

2. Magnetophoretic Forces

A magnetic dipole in a homogeneous magnetic field is not transported; because equal and opposite forces act on the N and S pole of the dipole, the body can only be rotated into an orientation of minimum energy. This is illustrated in Fig. 1A. The situation is more complicated when the field is nonhomogeneous, since then the body tends to move. The potential energy of a magnetic dipole with moment m in a magnetic field of strength H is $M \cdot H$. In general, the dipole will tend to move in the field to decrease this potential energy. If the dipole in Fig. 1A, fully rotated into the minimum-energy orientation, is located in the spreading field of Fig. 1B, the energy will still be smaller if the body is moved toward the pointed pole piece of

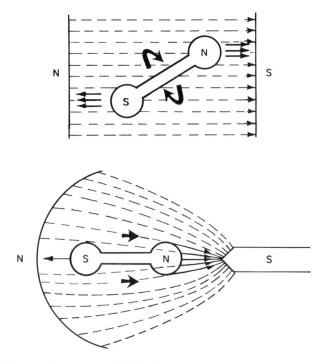

Figure 1. Forces acting on magnetic dipoles in magnetic fields. (A) Resultant rotational force in a homogeneous field; (B) resultant translational force in a nonuniform field.

the magnet. The force tending to move the dipole is given in general by the gradient of the potential energy:

$$F = \tfrac{1}{2} \int \nabla M \cdot H \, dv \tag{3}$$

where the force is integrated over the whole volume of the magnetized body.

Ferromagnetic materials are characterized by large values of magnetization in ordinary applied fields, saturation of magnetization at relatively low values of the applied field, and the existence of a temperature, the Curie point, above which these properties vanish. These properties are understood to be due to the existence of small regions in the material with typical volumes of 10^{-15} cm^3, within which all the atomic magnetic dipoles are aligned in parallel. The ferromagnetic body will have zero magnetic moment only if these regions, called magnetic domains (Weiss, 1907), are aligned randomly with respect to each other. In iron, magnetization occurs when domains which are already aligned in the direction of an applied field grow in size by accretion of neighboring domains which are misaligned. Because this growth is only partly reversible, there is a remanent magnetization when the external field is removed.

The ease by which this process of magnetization can occur varies with the size of the ferromagnetic body. It cannot occur at all in particles of the size of the domains themselves. Single-domain particles, then, can be expected to display unique properties in a magnetic field. These properties are useful in magnetophoretic cell separation.

If the single-domain particles, of about 0.1 μm or smaller, are suspended in a compliant medium such as a gel, they will be free to rotate in a magnetic field and will also be affected by Brownian motion, readily tending to random orientations in the absence of the field. Such a gel will have the ferromagnetic properties of a Curie point, large magnetization, and saturation, but will not display a remanent magnetization when the external field is zero. Such a gel is termed "superparamagnetic" (Bean and Livingston, 1959). This property would be displayed by soft gel beads with many single-domain particles embedded in them which can rotate within the bead. These superparamagnetic beads would show no mutual attraction and resultant clumping, in contrast to single-particle beads each containing a single-domain particle.

If we consider only the distance in the X direction in Fig. 2, and arrange the field in the X direction to increase proportionally with x, the force on a particle in the X direction is

$$F_x = \tfrac{1}{2} V H_x (dM/dx) + \tfrac{1}{2} V M (dH_x/dx) \tag{4}$$

by integrating equation (3) holding H_x and M constant over the volume of

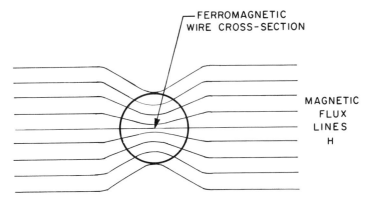

Figure 2. Concentration of the magnetic field in the vicinity of a ferromagnetic wire placed in a homogeneous applied field, leading to a strong local nonuniformity.

the particle; then differentiating. In a single-domain particle, the magnetization is a constant property of the material and is the same as the saturation magnetization of a multidomain sample, M_s, of that material. In this case,

$$F_x = \frac{1}{2} VM_s \,(dH_x/dx) \tag{5}$$

The force is therefore not dependent on the applied field, but only on the volume of the particle and on the gradient (dH_x/dx). In practice, larger gradients are obtainable when the field itself is large.

If, however, the particle is paramagnetic or is made of an assembly of domains as in the cases of ferromagnetic or superparamagnetic particles, then

$$M = H\chi \tag{6}$$

In this case M depends on the applied field but is a material property. Then, from equation (4)

$$F_x = VH\chi(dH_x/dx). \tag{7}$$

The force on these types of particles is linearly related to both the gradient of the applied field and to its magnitude. Magnetophoresis is facilitated by large nonhomogeneous fields.

Usually the magnetization of a ferromagnetic material is described by the permeability μ instead of the susceptibility χ. The two are simply related:

$$\mu = 1 + \rho\chi \tag{8}$$

where ρ is the density of the material.

Finally, it is useful to point out that two magnetic dipoles, aligned along their dipolar axes with respect to each other, separated by a distance much larger than their sizes, exert a force on each other given by

$$F = M^2 V^2 / 4\pi\mu_0 D^4 \qquad (9)$$

B. Previous Examples

1. Magnetic Separation of Cells

Only recently has magnetic attraction been used to separate cells, although magnetic separators have been in use in ore refining and other manufacturing applications for many years. As described above, a magnetic field can cause small magnetic particles to migrate only if it is nonhomogeneous; a uniform field only causes them to rotate (Fig. 1A). For example, certain flagellate bacteria found in salt marshes have chains of iron particles inside them, which orientate the cells when a uniform exterior magnetic field is applied. The cells do not actually migrate unless the flagellae are operating, when they display magnetotactism (Blakemore, 1975).

Magnetic particles are readily introduced into phagocytotic cells. Commercial preparations are available with magnetite particles coated with sensitizing agents such as polylysine, polybrene, polyarginine, or other basic polypeptides (Lichtenstein, 1973). When incubated in a mixture of blood cells under conditions which support phagocytosis, the phagocytes become magnetized and can be removed by passage through tubing located in a nonhomogeneous magnetic field obtained in the apparatus described in Section II.A.3.

Another method of cell separation has been derived from the field of high-gradient magnetic separation (HGMS) (Oberteuffer, 1974). It has been found that it is feasible to separate weakly magnetized cells, such as deoxygenated erythrocytes, provided that the magnetic field gradient is made high enough by placing fine stainless steel wires between the pole pieces of a homogeneous magnet. The wires have the effect of collecting the lines of force in the field, making small centers of attraction about them (Fig. 2). When the weakly magnetized cells are introduced, they are attracted to the wires and cover them. Melville et al. (1975) found that a homogeneous field of only 1.7 tesla was needed if the wires were 25 μm thick. In his arrangement, a 40-ml volume was packed with 1 ml of the wire. When whole ACD human blood flowed through the separator at 10^{-1} m/s for 1 h, 70% of the erythrocytes were retained in the magnet. A few cells either were hemolyzed or "leaked" through during the early forerun.

HGMS was also demonstrated by Owen (1978) with paramagnetic

human erythrocytes containing methemoglobin by treatment with sodium nitrite. In these experiments a superconducting magnet was used with a field of 3.3 tesla. The solenoid was packed with 40-μm No. 410 stainless steel wire. Only 2% of the cells treated in this way were eluted from the magnet, whereas 92% of reduced oxygenated cells were eluted. In a 50–50 mixture, 46% were retained. Although the higher magnetic field of the superconducting magnet allowed greater flow rates, it was driven well below its optimum field. Further, data on the effectiveness and efficiency of the separation as a function of cell loading is lacking, so it is not clear whether the system was demonstrated below or above its capacity— whether it might have been more efficient if run at a lower ratio of cells: wire surface.

2. Use of Magnetic Affinity Beads

It required considerable ingenuity to develop cell-specific separations from the above methods of magnetophoretic cell separation, operating on magnetized components of the cytoplasm. Because cell types have exquisitely specific receptors and other determinants on their surfaces, however, more general methods can be found, in which magnetic particles are attached to the outsides of cells. This was first reported for separations of surface-magnetized and fluorescent-labeled B lymphocytes from erythrocytes and from mixed spleen cells, including T lymphocytes (Molday et al., 1977). The separations from erythrocytes were remarkably effective: the retentate, bearing anti-immunoglobulin-coated beads, was 98% fluorescent, while the eluate was only 0.2 to 0.4% labeled. The separations from T lymphocytes were less effective: 76.4 to 81.6% fluorescent retentates and 1.4 to 3.0% fluorescent eluates, respectively. The method used for this separation was especially simple in which the cells were merely allowed to settle on a column of buffer placed near the pole of a permanent magnet for 2 h.

Obviously the technique of magnetizing the cells to be isolated is the key step in the procedure. This was achieved by preparing magnetic affinity beads of poly(methyl methacrylate–hydroxyethyl methacrylate–methacrylic acid) containing subdomain magnetite particles (Papell, 1965). Unfortunately, no information on the structure of these beads is available. From the details of the polymerization procedure, the beads must have polymerized from a mixed emulsion of the monomers and dispersed magnetite. It is not stated whether the beads are ferromagnetic or superparamagnetic, or whether they interact with each other.

It should be noted that the above magnetic affinity beads are not just coated magnetite, but contain at least 68 wt% polymer. These were selected from the more iron-rich, heavier products by sedimentation. The product yields are likely to be low, expensive, and uncertain, because both the beads and the subdomain particles on which they are based are minority products of the respective reactions from which they are made.

A more direct method of preparing single-domain magnetic microspheres for cell separation was described by Kronick et al. (1978). These beads were designed to balance magnetization against clumping. That is to say, particles which make cells to which they are attached easy to manipulate in a magnet also tend to attract each other and so tend to clump. It is desirable to maximize the force on the microspheres due to the external magnet. As seen in equation (5), this force increases with the volume of the magnetic particle. The forces among the particles, however, increase even more rapidly with the particle volume [equation (9)].

3. Designing a Magnetic Affinity Bead

Magnetic affinity microspheres for cell separation should have magnetic moments small enough so that they do not clump spontaneously before they interact with cells; the magnetic moments must, however, be large enough to provide magnetophoresis in the external magnetic field when they are attached to cells; the microspheres should be composed of a polymer which itself does not adhere nonspecifically to cells; and they should not be too difficult to prepare. In fact, compromises are usually made among these requirements.

Thermal motion is a dissociating influence acting on mutually attractive magnetic microspheres. In a suspension in which the energy of association is less than the thermal energy kT, the beads will diffuse apart. This attraction energy becomes lower when the polymer coatings around the magnetic particles are thicker, increasing the distance between the enclosed magnetic dipoles. From these considerations alone, it can be shown that the diameter D of the beads must be

$$D > (4\pi M^2/18\mu_0 kT)^{1/3} d^2 \qquad (10)$$

where M is the magnetization of the particle, μ_0 is the permeability of free space, and units are in the rationalized MKS system. From equation (10), it is seen that the required size of the nonclumping bead increases rapidly with that of the magnetic particle core d. If the maximum practical bead diameter is 2 μm, the equation specifies that the magnetic core diameter must be less than 50 nm.

Such a microsphere would have an iron content of 0.01%. An alternative structure could incorporate many magnetic subdomain or single-domain particles in each microsphere; if the particles were approximately spherical, such beads would be superparamagnetic and therefore would not clump at all, but would experience much greater forces in saturating magnetic fields than the single-particle microspheres described above. Such beads, however, have not yet been prepared as a uniform, characterized product.

The next requirement is that the cells, with beads attached, be able to be separated magnetophoretically. With the apparatus which is described below, this can be accomplished with the above beads with a migration speed of 2×10^{-2} cm/s. Using Stokes' law with equation (5), it can be calculated that 10-μm-diameter cells will be separated if they have only 10 beads attached.

A number of polymer formulations have been proposed for affinity microspheres for labeling cells which, unliganded, do not adhere nonspecifically to the cell surfaces. The products of "latex polymerization," beads of uniform size which form when polymers are prepared from emulsions, have been used in immunology for coagulation tests instead of the conventional red blood cells. In these tests, antibodies adsorbed on the surfaces of the beads cause them to attach to antigenic cell surfaces. While the resulting agglutination reaction is specific and sensitive, the beads also adsorb nonspecifically to cells when they are made from hydrophobic polymers: polystyrene or polymethyl methacrylate (Malin and Edwards, 1972; Milgrom and Goldstein, 1962). In addition, some antibody leaches from the beads, since the molecules are held by weak secondary forces. The problem of nonspecificity was overcome by Molday et al. (1974) and by Ljungstedt et al. (1978), who prepared beads from hydrogels such as poly(hydroxyethyl methacrylate) and polyacrylamide. ["Hydrogels" is the name given to insoluble water-swollen polymers, which have been found to have minimum interaction with tissue and blood cells in biocompatibility studies (Wichterle and Lim, 1960.)] When the hydrophilic hydrogel microbeads were chemically coupled to antibodies to cell-surface antigens, the beads adhered strongly to the cells. In the experiments described, no attempt was made to modulate the strength of the adhesion, which was maximized for purposes of demonstration. The strength of adhesion depends on both the degree of modification and the size of the beads, since stronger forces arising from shear are available at the bead–cell interface when the beads are large (Sell and An, 1971). [Interestingly, Ljungstedt et al. (1978) demonstrated that nonmagnetic microspheres could be used for cell separation by altering the cell density.]

We describe below a method for preparing magnetic microspheres from these nonspecifically adhering hydrogels, using the magnetite cores to initiate a polymer-forming reaction from the appropriate monomer on their surfaces (Kronick et al., 1978). In this reaction, ferrous ions dissolving from the surfaces of the particles react with persulfate in the solution to yield free radicals which initiate polymerization of the hydrogel:

$$Fe_3O_4 \xrightarrow{H^+} Fe^{2+}$$

$$Fe^{2+} + S_2O_8^{2-} \rightarrow Fe^{3+} + SO_4^{2-} + SO_4^-$$
$$SO_4^- + M \rightarrow SO_4M \cdot \xrightarrow{M} SO_4M(M_n)M \cdot$$

Since the reaction requires the ferrous ion at room temperature, it proceeds only in the vicinities of the particles containing this reagent.

4. Chemical Modification of Hydrogel Beads

Although hydrogel microbeads to label cells as described above is new (Molday *et al.,* 1974), the use of modified hydrogel surfaces in cell separation is an established batch technique. Convenient and straightforward methods for attaching proteins to hydrogels have been described. The most useful have been coupling of the amino groups to proteins or proteins to fixed carboxyl groups with the reagent l-ethyl-3-(3-dimethylaminopropyl) carbodiimide (Cuatrecasas and Parikh, 1972; Hoare and Koshland, 1967), attachment of amino groups of proteins to fixed hydroxyl groups by CNBr activation, and coupling of amino groups of proteins to fixed amino groups with glutaraldehyde (Weston and Avrameas, 1971). Fixed amino groups can be introduced into polyacrylamide by solvolysis with ethylene diamine or by degradation with alkaline hypochlorite (Schiller and Sven, 1956). This list of methods of modification is not complete, but includes those which we find to be most convenient for our purposes.

When proteins are fixed for affinity columns, the performance of the column is improved when a long "arm" is interposed between the protein and the substratum. The length of the arm is optimally 10 Å for this purpose. A convenient way of preparing the arm has been described by Cuatrecasas and Parikh (1972). After addition of 3,3'-diaminopropylamine to the fixed phase, the product is coupled to succinic anhydride. The terminal carboxylic acid of this product is finally coupled to N-hydroxysuccinimide in the presence of N,N'-dicyclohexylcarbodiimide. The final product is commercially available as the large beads used for affinity columns. It can be used to immobilize a variety of proteins under mild reaction conditions.

In the demonstration of cell labeling with antibody microbeads (Molday *et al.,* 1974), no arm was found to be necessary.

II. PROCEDURES

A. Preliminary

1. Preparation of Cells

Because this method depends on cell-surface determinants, it is desirable that the cells be prepared by techniques which do not change the pertinent chemistry of the surface. Standard methods are used for tissue and for cultured cells growing on plates: trypsin or collagenase, followed by incubation in calcium- and magnesium-free medium in a shaking or spinner flask overnight, so that the affected surface proteins can be regenerated. Obviously this incubation is unnecessary if the surface determinant is not a protein. After dispersal the suspension should be gently centrifuged or strained through sterile nylon mesh to remove clumps of cells.

2. Incubation with Magnetic Microspheres

One hundred times as many microspheres as cells to be separated are added to the cell suspension, which is then tumbled slowly end-over-end (30 rpm) for 30 min. The temperature depends on the type of cell, since affinity binding may be increased or decreased at 4°C with respect to room temperature (Rutishauser and Edelman, 1977). If the ligand is metabolically active, then the incubation should be done at 4°C to suppress the cell response. The tumbling incubation is carried out in sterile test tubes about $^{3}/_{4}$ full.

3. Magnetic Separation

The apparatus is shown in Fig. 3. The magnet is prepared from a commercially available electromagnet (Edmund Scientific Co., 1895 Edscorp Building, Barrington, N.J., Cat. No. 71936) by adding a 1.3-mm steel shim to cover the inner pole and then securing the armature plate with brass screws tapped into the outer pole around its circumference (Fig. 4). The field region which is used is in the groove which runs around the magnet between the outer pole and the armature plate. Small brass or aluminum strips are screwed to the outside of the magnet to hold a length of 1-mm i.d. × 1.7-mm o.d. plastic tubing in the groove in such a way that the tubing can easily be removed and replaced. The magnet is driven at about 2.5 A with a 6-V battery eliminator (for example, Canalco, Rockville, Md., Model 124).

The cells flow from a syringe barrel mounted slightly above the magnet through a sterile 3-way stopcock (Pharmaseal Inc., Toa Alta, Puerto Rico, Model K-75) and a length of plastic tubing wrapped in the groove of the magnet described above, and drop into sterile culture tubes or flasks (Fig. 3). The syringes have offset outlet holes so that cells and magnetic microspheres are not trapped in a pocket below the outlet. The tubing should be arranged without level stretches, to discourage the cells from settling. The collection tubes or flasks should be slanted on a rack or holder under the end of the outlet tubing, so that they can be quickly exchanged by hand. The whole apparatus can be centered on a single laboratory standard.

Before beginning the separation, the volume of liquid in the tubing

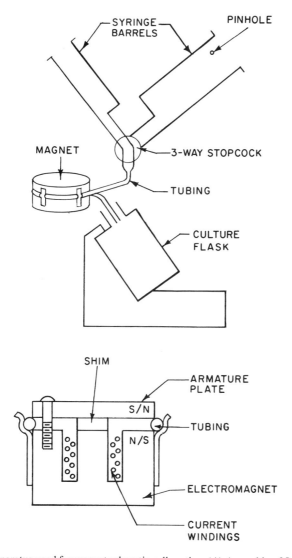

Figure 3.   Apparatus used for magnetophoretic cell sorting. (A) Assembly of flow system; (B) details of electromagnet separator (see text for dimensions).

from the stopcock to the outlet should be measured. This is easily done by mounting a 1-ml syringe filled with water to the filled stopcock and tubing, admitting an air bubble into the tubing from the other, empty, syringe, and measuring the volume of water from the filled syringe required to force the bubble to the outlet of the tubing. The syringes are used without their plungers in the separation procedure, but the plungers should be retained

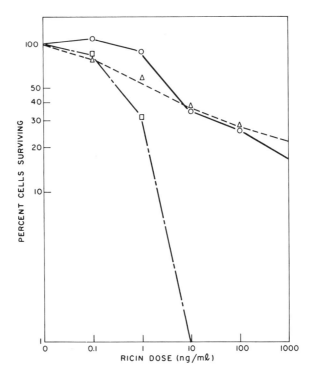

Figure 4. Protein synthesis in HeLa cells which have been challenged with various doses of ricin. Cells are incubated at 37°C overnight in Earle's minimum essential medium with 10% newborn calf serum and the doses of ricin shown in the figure. This medium is replaced with fresh medium containing no ricin but with 50 Curie ^{11}C-leu. After a 1-hr incubation at 37°C, the medium is removed; the cells, digested with NaOH; and the proteins, precipitated with 50% TCA. The precipitates are filtered and analyzed in a scintillation counter for ^{11}C uptake. (□— · —□) Ricin-sensitive retentate; (Δ – – – –Δ) R^{R}II cells, ricin resistant; and (O———O) eluate from 50:50 mixture of wild and resistant cells.

in sterile condition in case an air bubble is accidentally admitted to the line and impedes the flow. They can then be used to push the liquid through the tubing until the bubbles are eliminated. (A pinhole in the side of the syringe barrel near the top, which is closed with a fingertip when pushing the liquid through, allows the plunger to be withdrawn without pulling back the liquid in the tubing.)

B. Preparation of Single-Domain Magnetic Affinity Beads

1. Magnetic Microspheres

Hydroxyethyl methacrylate is distilled at 2 torr and 79°C; methacrylic acid, at 10 torr and 60.5°C. N,N'-methylenebisacrylamide is electrophoresis-grade, having been purified by repeated recrystallizations. Magnetite is a synthetic product used for magnetic recording, with a uniform particle size. That used in our preparations comprises cubical particles with 50-nm edges (Wright Industries, Brooklyn, N.Y.). Smaller particles (Papell, 1965), which are much more expensive, can also be used (Ferrofluidics Corp., Burlington, Vt.). Each batch should be washed several times with water and analyzed by emission spectroscopy for metal ions. A monomer mixture is first prepared, comprising, by weight, 70% hydroxyethyl methacrylate, 10% N,N'-methylenebisacrylamide, and 20% methacrylic acid.

Fifty milligrams of 50-nm magnetite particles and 50 mg of $Na_3P_2O_7$ are homogenized in 40 ml water. The suspension is homogenized with a high-speed homogenizer and sonicated in a 50-ml round flask under nitrogen. After adding 2 g of the monomer mixture, the pH is adjusted to 4. Then, 30 mg of $Na_2S_4O_8$ are added. A 100-μl sample is removed for analysis of dissolved monomer by determining its UV absorbance at 210 nm, after centrifuging away the magnetite (specific absorbance = $8 \times 10^{-4}\,cm^{-1}M^{-1}$). A stirrer and a nitrogen inlet and outlet are fitted to the flask, which is closed to the air. The stirrer should be a paddle conforming to the bottom of the flask, and should turn only fast enough to prevent the magnetite from settling on the bottom. The reaction, run with this slow stirring and flow of nitrogen, typically takes about 2 h at room temperature. At the end of this time, the flask is opened and a sample is again analyzed by UV absorbance at 210 mn. At least 80% of the monomer should have been consumed.

The magnetized product is placed in a 4-oz bottle and precipitated onto the side of the bottle by placing it against the edge of a pole of a large horseshoe magnet (e.g., Edmund Scientific Co., Barrington, N.J., Catalogue No. 70,810). The precipitation and resuspension in neutral buffer is repeated several times to wash the sample free of excess monomer and ungelled polymer: The neutral buffer facilitates this removal by swelling the polyelectrolyte gel. Typically it may take several hours for each precipitation, working with 50-ml volumes in a 0.3-tesla magnet.

Three 2-ml samples of the washed product are removed to tared crucibles and dried at 110°C to constant weight to determine the yield on a dry weight-to-suspension volume basis. The crucibles are then ignited free of organic matter in a furnace or on a Mecker burner to determine the inorganic content as Fe_2O_3, obtaining constant weights by conventional gravimetric technique. The product should also be examined by electron microscopy to determine particle sizes; the suspension should be sonicated immediately before mounting on the microscope grid or stub, to avoid artifacts due to clumping.

Magnetic microspheres consisting of albumin spheres from 0.2- to 2-μm diameter containing 10- to 20-nm magnetite particles were used for drug delivery (Widder *et al.*, 1978). These were prepared from a reversed emulsion of albumin–magnetite–water in cottonseed oil, heating at 120°–140°C to harden them. The product was spheres with a distribution of sizes, the magnetite being concentrated at the peripheries of the beads. They could be retained in blood flowing at 0.5 cm/s with a 0.8-tesla magnet.

2. Derivatives

A mixture of 250 mg (dry weight) of beads, 0.1 g diaminoheptane, and 100 mg 1-ethyl-3-(3-dimethylaminopropyl) carbodiimide in 15 ml of 10 mM phosphate buffer at pH 5.0 is shaken with 5-mm glass beads for 5 h at 4°C. In this reaction the carboxyl groups of methacrylic acid are amidated with the diamine, introducing an arm with an available amino group for attachment of ligands.

A fluorescent label is next applied to a portion of the free amino groups. The above product (250 mg dry weight) is precipitated and washed magnetically four times and resuspended in 170 ml of 10 mM sodium borate buffer at pH 8.5. To this is added 0.140 g fluorescein isothiocyanate in 1 ml alcohol. A few 5-mm glass beads are added, and the reaction mixture is shaken at room temperature for 3 h. The microspheres are precipitated magnetically and washed with neutral buffer until there is no detectable free dye.

To activate the beads for coupling to proteins, 250 mg (dry weight) of the above fluorescent product containing free amino groups is suspended in 15 ml of 10 mM phosphate buffer at pH 7, containing 1% distilled glutaraldehyde. The suspension is shaken with glass beads for 2 h at room temperature.

The suspension is at this point sterile. It can be precipitated and washed as above with sterile neutral phosphate buffer and stored for several months in the cold as a sterile product. It is important that Tris buffer not come into contact with this intermediate, since it would react with the active aldehyde centers. To attach ligands, typically 1 mg of sterile protein is added to 50 mg (dry weight) of the activated microspheres in 2 ml of 10-mM phosphate buffer at pH 6.9–7.0. The suspension is shaken at 4°C overnight and washed free of excess protein by repeated magnetic precipitations. If the ligand is stable enough (for example, the lectin ricin or some short polypeptides), the beads can be sterilized after its attachment by suspension in 60% alcohol, precipitation, and resuspension in sterile phosphate buffered saline.

The capacity of the microspheres to bind proteins is best determined for each ligand. This requires labeling the ligand, either with radioactive iodine, ^{14}C, ^{3}H, etc., or with a fluorescent label. It must also be established that the labeling does not interfere with the binding to the microspheres. The reaction mixture described above for attaching ligands is prepared in a series of 1-ml Eppendorff centrifuge tubes, containing different amounts of labeled protein, including zero protein in the control and 1 mg/ml with no microspheres in a blank. At least 4 tubes are prepared at each protein concentration. The reaction is allowed to proceed as described, tumbling the reaction tubes end-over-end. Samples are taken at about 1, 2, 5, and 18 h by spinning down the appropriate tubes, removing the supernatant, and determining the amount of label in it. If radioactive iodine is used, the tubes containing the pelleted microspheres can be placed directly in a γ-ray counter.

If the ligand cannot be analyzed in this way, it is useful to determine the capacity of the microspheres for protein in a general way by measuring their uptake of cytochrome c. The absorbance of a solution of 4×10^{-6} M cytochrome c solution in 5 mM phosphate buffer at pH 7.0 is measured at the Soret peak (410 nm for fully oxidized cytochrome; 402 nm for reduced).Ten milligrams of activated microspheres are precipitated in each of two 15-ml test tubes. Eight milliliters of the cytochrome c solution are added to one of the test tubes, and 4 ml of buffer followed by 4 ml of cytochrome c solution are added to the other. The microspheres are resuspended; the tubes are capped and tumbled overnight at 4°C. After the reaction, each tube is centrifuged, the contents are diluted 4 times, and the absorbance is determined at the same wavelength as previously. From this data the uptake of cytochrome c can be calculated for each sample.

III. EXAMPLES

A. Toxic Lectins

This category comprises a number of dimeric proteins which bind to specific carbohydrate receptors on the cell surface and influence the cell metabolism. Included are the dimeric proteins ricin from *Ricinus communis* L., abrin from *Abrus precatorius,* modeccin from *Adenia digitata,* diphtheria toxin, and choleragen. All of these are believed to act on cells by first binding and then dissociating into a pair of polypeptides—a haptomer, with a specific binding site, and an effectomer, which interacts with the cell metabolism. In most cases (Olsnes and Pihl, 1976) the polypeptide pairs can be dissociated synthetically to yield free haptomer and effectomer. The free haptomer binds specifically as does the intact lectin, but has no toxic effect; the free effectomers influence the biochemistry of cell-free systems but cannot enter intact cells. If an integral lectin is used as a ligand for microspheres, the suspension must be carefully washed to remove free toxin, which typically is active at picomolar levels. The following examples were carried out under these conditions.

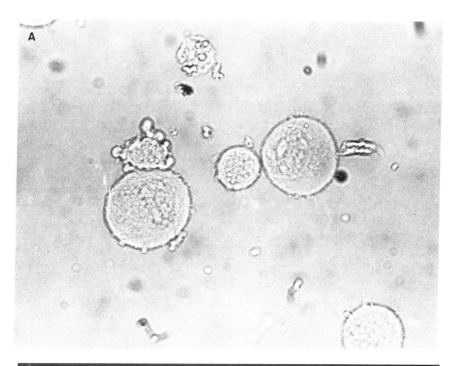

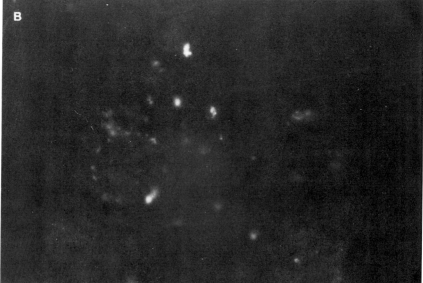

Figure 5. Competition of free ganglioside G_{M1} with C-1300 neuroblastoma cells for magnetic microspheres with choleragen ligand. (A) Cells which have been incubated with fluorescent choleragen-coated microspheres, viewed in light field; (B) same as (A), dark-field fluorescence;

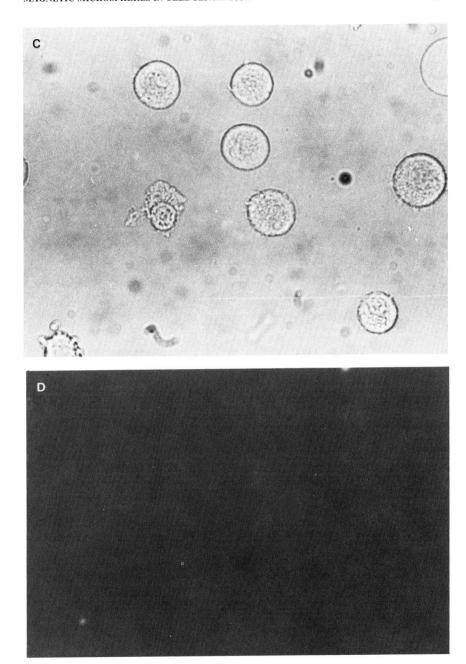

(C) cells which had been labeled with G_{MI} were incubated with choleragen-coated magnetic microspheres in the presence of excess G_{MI} and viewed in light field; (D) same as (C), dark field. The binding of the microspheres is inhibited.

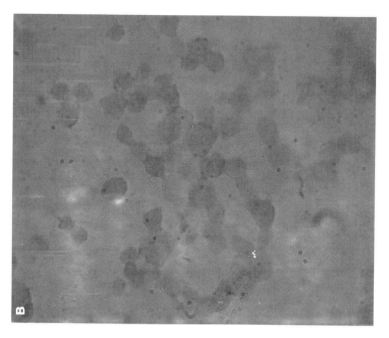

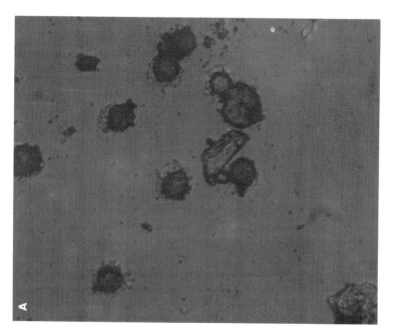

Figure 6. C-1300 neuroblastoma cells after having been sorted and incubated for 24 h, stained with HRP-conjugated choleragen. (A) Cells binding microspheres and retained in the magnetic field (choleragen-positive cells); (B) cells not binding microspheres and not retained in the magnetic field (choleragen-negative cells).

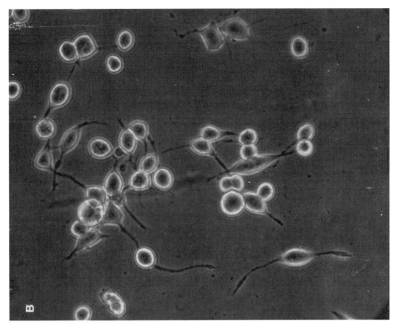

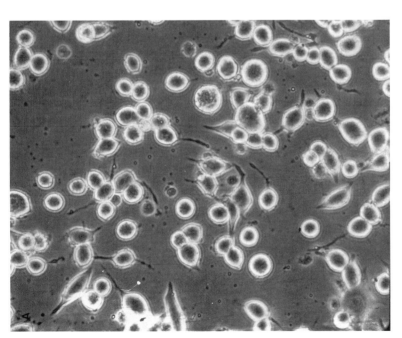

Figure 7. Neuroblastoma cells grown for 3 days after magnetophoretic sorting. (A) Eluate, G_{M1}-negative; (B) retentate, G_{M1}-positive.

1. Ricin- and Abrin-Resistant HeLa Cells*

Ricin is a water-soluble glycoprotein isolated from beans of *Ricinus communis* L. (Olsnes and Pihl, 1976). It has a molecular weight of 65,000 daltons and binds with a dissociation constant of about 10^{-9} M to terminal galactose residues. It also binds free galactose with a dissociation constant of 7×10^{-5} M (Olsnes *et al.*, 1974). When HeLa cells are grown in the presence of graded amounts of a lectin, strains exhibiting various levels of resistivity to its toxic effects can be selected and cloned. In this example we worked with the line $R^R II$, cloned by Fodstad *et al.* (1977), and described by Sandvig *et al.* (1978), which has only 20% of the number of ricin receptors, on the average, as the wild cells.

Monolayer cultures of wild and ricin-resistant HeLa cells were suspended by treating with trypsin using conventional techniques. After having been washed free of debris, they were suspended at 4×10^5 cells/ml in Earle's minimum essential medium containing 10% newborn calf serum and shaken in a CO_2-controlled atmosphere at 37°C for 2 h.

To determine the proper amounts of reagents to use, preliminary experiments were run with wild cells and various amounts of beads, and with beads carrying various amounts of ligand. These experiments were evaluated first by counting fluorescent-labeled cells under a fluorescence microscope. From the preliminary experiments it was seen that the minimum amount of ricin which was effective as a ligand for the wild cells was applied to the beads from a mixture of ricin and bovine serum albumin in the ratio of 0.20 mg/ml to 0.1 mg/ml. Lower ratios gave many cells which were free of beads. It was also seen, and confirmed by magnetic precipitation experiments, that 1.25 mg/ml (dry weight) of beads in the cell suspension was an adequate amount, resulting in few clumps. The amount of ricin on the microspheres was, by ^{125}I-γ-ray analysis, 0.11 mg/ml. The microspheres with ligand were sterilized by suspension for 1 h in 60% alcohol; they were then gently centrifuged and resuspended in sterile medium containing no protein.

60% alcohol was placed in the syringes of the magnetophoretic separation apparatus (Fig. 3), run through to the outlet of the tubing, and held for 30 min. The syringes were emptied to the stopcock and loaded with sterile medium containing no protein, which was used to displace the alcohol in the tubing by again emptying the syringes down to the stopcock. Into the sample syringe was then placed 5 ml of medium containing 10% newborn calf serum, cells and beads; into the other, 10 ml of medium with

---

*This section was written with Sjur Olsnes, Norsk Hydros Institute for Cancer Research, Oslo, Norway.

serum, anti-ricin immunoglobulin, and 20 mM lactose, which is a competitive substrate for ricin binding (Sandvig *et al.*, 1976). The system was
designed to first separate the wild cells, most of which bind ricin, from the
resistant ones, which bind less; then to free the wild cells from the microspheres; and then to inactivate all free and immobilized ricin with the
antibody.

With the magnet on, the cells were run through the system at about 4
sec/drop and flushed with 5 ml of medium containing serum, collecting in a
sterile culture flask. The magnet was turned off, and the retained cells were
washed out with the contents of the second syringe, containing serum,
antibody, and lactose.

Additional medium with serum was added to the culture flasks and the
cells were incubated for 2 weeks. They were then tested for sensitivity to
ricin. The results are shown in Fig. 4. The dose–response curve for the
eluate is identical to that for the starting ricin-resistant cells, designated by
Fodstad *et al.* (1977) as $R^R II$, and very different from the sensitive retentate. Less than 10% of the eluted cells were of the sensitive type.

2. Membrane Ganglioside G_{M1}

The ganglioside content of cell membranes is correlated with properties of cell growth (Hakomori, 1975; Hollenberg *et al.*, 1974), differentiation (De Baeque *et al.*, 1976; Stein-Douglas *et al.*, 1976), and transformation. Sensitive methods for the detection of the ganglioside G_{M1} have been
developed utilizing the preferential affinity of choleragen (cholera enterotoxin) for this molecule (Cuatrecasas, 1973; Hollenberg *et al.*, 1974).

Variations in ganglioside content have been investigated in solid
tumors, derived cell lines and cell hybrids (Yogeeswaran *et al.*, 1973). An
example is C-1300 neuroblastoma, a neuroectodermally derived transplantable tumor with the potential of expressing differentiated functions *in vitro*
(Graham *et al.*, 1974). Recently it was noted that a clone of this tumor
grown *in vitro* demonstrated individual heterogeneity in the cell surface
expression of G_{M1} as indicated by the binding of either horseradish peroxidase (HRP)-conjugated or fluorescein-conjugated choleragen.

One milligram of choleragen (Schwarz/Mann, Orangeburg, N.Y.) was
attached to 50 mg of activated microspheres in 2 ml of 5 mM phosphate at
pH 7.0, shaking with glass beads at 4°C for 24 h. The modified beads were
washed by centrifugation and resuspension 3 times into phosphate-buffered
saline (PBS).

Single-cell suspensions of C-1300 neuroblastoma cells grown to con-
fluency were used for these studies. $2–5 \times 10^6$ cells were incubated with
0.1–1.0 mg (dry wt.) of choleragen-conjugated magnetic microspheres at

4°C for 30 min. To facilitate the removal of unbound microspheres the cell suspension was layered on top of fetal calf serum and centrifuged at 800g for 10 min. This procedure was repeated twice. The cells were resuspended in 2 ml of Dulbecco's BME for the separation procedure. Inhibition of binding of the choleragen-conjugated microspheres could be demonstrated by preincubating the cells with purified G_{MI} (30 mg/ml) in 1 ml of Dulbecco's BME at 4°C for 30 min. The microspheres were then added to the cell suspension in the presence of G_{MI}. G_{MI} was purified by thin-layer chromatography after isolation of whole-brain gangliosides as described by Lauter and Trams (1962).

Two milliliters of a cell suspension which contained labeled microspheres was passed by gravity flow through 1.0-mm polyvinyl chloride tubing wound 6 times around the circumferential edges of the pole pieces of a 12-inch electromagnet rather than that in Fig. 3. The spread of the field across these edges was 0.1 tesla/cm from 1 tesla. Various flow rates were used, from 0.3 ml/min to 3 ml/min. After the eluted fraction of cells was collected with the magnetic field on, the tubing was washed with medium into the eluted fraction. Then the magnetic field was turned off, and the retentate was washed through with more medium and collected separately as a single fraction.

The binding of choleragen to neuroblastoma cells can be demonstrated using HRP-choleragen, fluorescein-conjugated choleragen, or choleragen-conjugated fluorescent magnetic beads. The results of all three techniques show that only 10–20% of the neuroblastoma cells bind cholera toxin. Specificity has been demonstrated by the inhibition of the binding with ganglioside G_{MI}. Figures 5a and 5b show the presence of fluorescent magnetic beads on the surfaces of the cells after they were incubated together. Figures 5c and 5d show the inhibition of this binding by G_{MI} in the incubation mixture, even after the cells have been preincubated with ganglioside G_{MI}.

To demonstrate the effectiveness of the cell separation, aliquots from both the retained and eluted samples were plated out onto a glass coverslip and incubated *in vitro* for 24 h. Each coverslip was then stained with HRP-conjugated choleragen (Graham and Karnovsky, 1966). Figure 6 shows the result of this procedure for an unfractionated sample, the retained portion and the eluted portion. The two unfractionated samples contained 12.5 and 15.0% of choleragen-positive cells, whereas the retained and eluted fractions contained 99.0% and 99.5%, or 1.0% and 1.5%, respectively. Figure 7 shows the morphology of the two populations 3 days after separation. They have flattened to the culture plate and continue to grow. We cannot demonstrate specific morphological differences between the two populations.

B. Antibody Ligands

1. Brain Cells

The development of brain tissue involves the elaboration of myelin by oligodendrocytes, which are difficult to separate from the other cells in studies of the process. Since these cells express specific proteins, however, they are suited for isolation by means of magnetophoresis with microspheres conjugated with an antibody against them. In this example (Campbell *et al.*, 1978) an indirect antibody technique was used, in which rat brain oligodendrocytes are labeled with rabbit antibody, and are then bound to magnetic microspheres bearing goat anti-rabbit immunoglobulin.

Brain cells were isolated from 10-day-old rats and enriched with the glial fraction (Campbell *et al.*, 1977). The suspension was incubated with rabbit serum against bovine oligodendrocytes and washed. The cells were incubated with magnetic microspheres bearing the above ligand for 30 min at 4°C and centrifuged on fetal calf serum at $800g$ for 10 min. They were then passed through apparatus similar to that in Fig. 4, except that the magnet was the 12-inch electromagnet described in Section III.A.3. The tubing was fastened to the edge of the pole piece during the collection of immunonegative cells, and removed for collection of the retentate. Oligodendrocytes were identified by scanning and transmission electron microscope examination. These cells, from 5–8 μm in diameter with high nucleus:cytoplasm ratio and occasionally attached to myelin fragments, comprised over 90% of the retentate. Further confirmation of their identity was their extension of processes within 1 h of incubation at 37°C on coverslips coated with succinylated polylysine.

REFERENCES

Bean, C. P., and Livingston, J. D., 1959, Superparamagnetism, *J. Appl. Phys. Suppl.* **30**:1205.

Blakemore, R., 1975, Magnetotactic bacteria, *Science* **190**:377.

Campbell, G. LeM., Schachner, M., and Sharrow, S. W., 1977, Isolation of glial cell enriched and depleted populations from mouse cerebellum by density gradient centrifugation and electronic cell sorting, *Brain Res.* **127**:69.

Campbell, G. LeM., Abramsky, O., and Silberberg, D., 1978, Isolation of oligodendrocytes from mouse cerebellum using magnetic microspheres, *Society for Neuroscience Abstracts* **4**:64.

Cuatrecasas, P., 1973, Interaction of *Vibrio cholerae* enterotoxin with cell membranes, *Biochemistry,* **12**:3547.

Cuatrecasas, P., and Parikh, I., 1972, Adsorbents for affinity chromatography. Use of *N*-hydroxysuccinimide esters of agarose, *Biochemistry* **11**:2291.

De Baeque, C., Johnson, A. B., Naiki, M., Schwarting, G. A., and Marcus, D. M., 1976, Ganglioside localisation in cerebellar cortex: An immunoperoxidase study with antibody to G_{M1} ganglioside, *Brain Res.* **114**:117.

Fodstad, Ø., Olsnes, S., and Pihl, A., 1977, Inhibitory effect of abrin and ricin on the growth of transplantable murine tumors and of abrin on human cancers in nude mice, *Cancer Res.* **37**:4559.

Graham, R. C., and Karnovsky, M. J., 1966, The early stages of absorption of injected horse-radish peroxidase in the proximal tubules of mouse kidney: Ultrastructural cytochemistry by a new technique, *J. Histochem. Cytochem.* **14**:291.

Graham, D. I., Gonatas, N. D., and Charalampous, F. C., 1974, The undifferentiated and extended forms of C-1300 murine neuroblastoma: Ultrastructural studies and detection of lectin binding sites, *Amer. J. Pathol.* **76**:285.

Hakomori, S., 1975, Structure and organization of cell surface glycolipids: Dependency on cell growth and malignant transformation, *Biochim. Biophys. Acta* **417**:55.

Hoare, D. G., and Koshland, D. E., 1967, A quantitative method for the quantitative modifi-cation and estimation of carboxylic acid groups in proteins, *J. Biol. Chem.* **242**:2447.

Hollenberg, M. D., Fishman, P. H., Bennett, V., and Cuatrecasas, P., 1974, Cholera toxin and cell growth: Role of membrane gangliosides, *Proc. Natl. Acad. Sci. USA* **71**:4224.

Kronick, P. L., Campbell, G. LeM., and Joseph, K., 1978, Magnetic microspheres prepared by redox polymerization used in a cell separation based on gangliosides, *Science* **200**:1074.

Lauter, K. J., and Trams, G., 1962, Isolation and characterization of gangliosides, *Biochim. Biophys. Acta* **60**:350.

Lichtenstein, B., 1973, Method and apparatus for lymphocyte separation from blood, U.S. Patent No. 3,709,791 (Jan. 9, 1973).

Ljungstedt, I., Eckman, B., and Sjöholm, I., 1978, Detection and separation of lymphocytes with specific surface receptors, by using microparticles, *Biochem. J.* **170**:161.

Malin, S. F., and Edwards, J., 1972, Detection of hepatitis associated antigen by latex agglu-tination, *Nature New Biol. (London)* **2350**:182.

Melville, D., Paul, F., and Roath, S., 1975, Direct magnetic separation of red cells from whole blood, *Nature (London)* **255**:706.

Milgrom, F., and Goldstein, R., 1962, Agglutination of sensitized red blood cells by latex particles, *Vox Sang.* **7**:86.

Molday, R. S., Dreyer, W., Rembaum, A., and Yen, S. P. S., 1974, Latex spheres as markers for studies of cell surface receptors by SEM, *Nature (London)* **249**:81.

Molday, R. S., Yen, S. P. S., and Rembaum, A., 1977, Application of magnetic microspheres in labelling and separation of cells, *Nature (London)* **268**:437.

Oberteuffer, J. O., 1974, Magnetic separation: A review of principles, devices, and applica-tions, *IEEE Trans. Magn.* **10**(2):223.

Olsnes, S., and Pihl, A., 1976, Abrin, ricin, and their associated agglutinins, in *Receptors and Recognition Series B: The Specificity and Action of Animal, Bacterial and Plant Toxins,* (P. Cuatrecasas, ed.), pp. 130–173, Chapman and Hall, London.

Olsnes, S., Saltvedt, E., and Pihl, A., 1974, Isolation and comparison of galactose-binding lectins from *Abrus precatorius* and *Ricinus communis, J. Biol. Chem.* **249**:803.

Owen, C., 1978, High gradient magnetic separation of erythrocytes, *Biophys. J.* **22**:171.

Papell, S. S., 1965, Low-viscosity magnetic fluid obtained by the colloidal suspension of mag-netic particles, U. S. Patent 3,215,572.

Rutishauser, U. S., and Edelman, G. M., 1977, Fractionation and manipulation of cells with chemically modified fibers and surfaces, in *Methods of Cell Separation* (N. Catsimpoolas, ed.), Vol. 1, p. 204, Plenum Press, New York.

Sandvig, K., Olsnes, S., and Pihl, A., 1976, Kinetics of binding of the toxic lectins abrin and ricin to surface receptors of human cells. *J. Biol. Chem.* **254**:3977.

Sandvig, K., Olsnes, S., and Pihl, A., 1978, Binding uptake and degradation of the toxic proteins abrin and ricin by toxin-resistant cell variants, *Eur. J. Biochem.* **82**:13.

Schiller, A. M., and Sven, T. J., 1956, Ionic derivatives of polyacrylamide, *Ind. Eng. Chem.* **48**:2132.

Sell, S., and An, T., 1971, Studies on rabbit lymphocytes *in vitro*. XIV. Fractionation of rabbit peripheral blood lymphocytes by antibody-coated polyacrylamide beads, *J. Immunol.* **197**:1302.

Stein-Douglas, K., Schwarting, G. A., Naiki, M., and Marcus, D. M., 1976, Gangliosides as markers for murine lymphocyte subpopulations, *J. Exp. Med.* **143**:822.

Weiss, P., 1907, L'Hypothèse du champ moléculaire et la propriété ferromagnétique, *J. Phys.* **6**:661.

Weston, P. D., and Avrameas, S., 1971, Proteins coupled to polyacrylamide beads using glutaraldehyde, *Biochem. Biophys. Res. Commun.* **45**:1574.

Wichterle, O., and Lim, D., 1960, Hydrophilic gels for biological use, *Nature* (London) **185**:117.

Widder, K. J., Senyei, A. E., and Scarpelli, D. G., 1978, Magnetic microspheres: A model system for site specific drug delivery *in vivo*, *Proc. Soc. Exp. Biol. Med.* **58**:141.

Yogeeswaran, G., Murray, R. K. Pearson, M. L., Sanwal, B. D., McMorris, F. A., and Ruddle, F. H., 1973, Glycosphingolipids of clonal lines of mouse neuroblastoma × L-cell hybrids, *J. Biol. Chem.* **248**:1231.

4

Isolation of Human Blood Phagocytes by Counterflow Centrifugation Elutriation

FABIAN J. LIONETTI, STEPHEN M. HUNT, AND C. ROBERT VALERI

I. INTRODUCTION

The principle of cell separation by counterflow centrifugation was first enunciated by Lindahl (1948) who derived an equation defining the position of particles in a centrifugal field opposed by fluid flowing in the centripetal direction. He designed a "counterstreaming" centrifuge which concentrated yeast particles in planes of equilibrium dependent upon the radius and density of the yeast and the viscosity and density of the medium (Lindahl, 1956). In an early study with the "counterstreaming" centrifuge eosinophilic leukocytes from horse blood were concentrated and the final cell suspension contained 20–30% (Lindahl and Lindahl, 1955). A significant advance was made by McEwen et al. (1968) who designed rotors for use with a standard preparative centrifuge. Their studies were largely responsible for the production of the simple equipment which makes counterflow cell separation generally available. Polystyrene microspheres, yeasts, plant, and blood cells were resolved into subpopulations with diameters which ranged from 0–20 μm. In the first attempts to isolate leukocytes, whole blood with a ratio of 700 red cells to 1 leukocyte was concentrated to a ratio of 4:1. In a sample of whole blood in which 73% of the white cells consisted of granulocytes, counterflow centrifugation recovered 94% of them in the separation chambers. With a prototype rotor designed

FABIAN J. LIONETTI AND STEPHEN M. HUNT • Center for Blood Research, Boston, Massachusetts 02115.   C. ROBERT VALERI • Naval Blood Research Laboratory, Boston University Medical Center, Boston, Massachusetts 02118.

later, McEwen *et al.* (1971) achieved 99% recovery of leukocytes from malaria-infected monkey blood. The fragile parasite-infected erythrocytes remained in suspension during the separation of leukocytes, preventing the disruptive physical trauma due to packing that would normally occur with conventional centrifugation. Over the past few years improvements in the design of separation chambers used in the rotor have been made (Grabske, 1978; Sanderson *et al.*, 1976; Sanderson and Bird, 1977) and it is now possible to achieve quantitative isolation of granulocytes from 10–20 ml of whole blood or buffy coat containing only 1% of mononuclear cells and as little as 2% red cells (Lionetti *et al.*, 1977; Persidsky and Olson, 1978).

II. ISOLATION OF GRANULOCYTES FROM HUMAN BLOOD

In human blood red cells outnumber leukocytes in the ratio 800 to 1 and platelets by a ratio of 50 to 1. The specific gravity of leukocytes ($\approx$1.07) is higher than plasma ($\approx$1.03) and platelets ($\approx$1.04) but less than erythrocytes ($\approx$1.09). Thus, leukocytes subjected to a gravitational force sediment as the buffy coat interface between plasma and red cells. That they are found in a sedimented or centrifuged blood sample positioned between plasma and packed red cells indicates white cells do not settle in conformity with Stokes' law* by which the sedimentation velocity of rigid spheres is markedly influenced by size as it depends on the square of their radii. Granulocytes whose radii in suspension are larger (4–5 μm) than red cells (3–3.5 μm) would be expected to settle to the bottom of the tube. They actually do settle fastest when whole blood is extensively diluted (Persidsky and Olson, 1978), a condition that prevails in the counterflow centrifuge. When granulocytes are subjected to hydrodynamic forces generated by the counterflow of medium in the centripetal direction, conditions at equilibrium are those in which density and viscosity effects are significantly reduced and blood cell separations show a greater dependence on size. Thus, by appropriate selection of media, flow rates, and centrifugal forces, granulocytes may be resolved from platelets, red cells, and lymphocytes. Furthermore, if the mononuclear cells are separated previously from leukocytes by gradient centrifugation with Ficoll–Hypaque, lymphocytes with radii of 2.5–3.0 μm may be separated from monocytes with radii of 4–5 μm by coun-

---

*According to Stokes' Law, the sedimentation velocity of rigid spheres is given by:

$$S.V. = \frac{2}{9} \frac{r^2 (p - p^1)g}{\eta}$$

where $S.V.$ = sedimentation velocity, r = radius of the particle, p and p^1 = densities of particle and medium respectively, η = viscosity of the medium, and g = gravity.

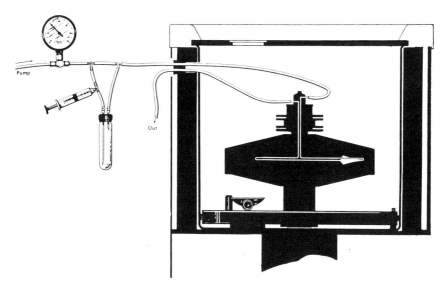

FIGURE 1. Schematic drawing of the counterflow centrifuge. Buffers are pumped into the rotor from a reservoir through the tubing at left marked "pump." Blood or buffy coat is admitted with the syringe and mixed with buffer in the stoppered tube. Granulocytes are held in the white blood cell chamber within the rotor while red blood cells, lymphocytes, and platelets are flushed into an external receptacle, marked "out." After the run, the rotor is dismantled, and the collection chamber containing the isolated granulocytes is removed. Reprinted with permission from *Transfusion*.

terflow elutriation using incremental increases of flow rate through the elutriator rotor at successive time intervals (this chapter, Section III).

The elutriation system employing the Beckman JE-6 rotor is illustrated in Fig. 1. The chambers used for the separation of white cells in the Beckman rotor are shown in Fig. 2. Either may be mounted in the rotor, and for

FIGURE 2. Chambers for Beckman JE-6 rotor. Beckman chamber on the left has a distinct cell boundary that can be visualized with the aid of a synchronized stroboscopic lamp. The Sanderson design on the right permits finer resolution of similar cell types, i.e., mononuclear cells.

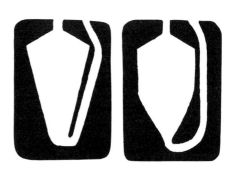

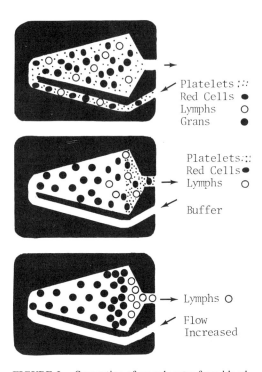

FIGURE 3. Separation of granulocytes from blood.

certain studies, two chambers may be used. An illustration of the separation of granulocytes from the other cell types in whole blood is shown if Fig. 3. To separate granulocytes using counterflow centrifugation, the following are needed: (a) a stationary harness through which blood or cell suspensions are injected through a valve using a syringe, (b) a mixing chamber in which cells and buffer are mixed, (c) a pump to force the cell suspension into and through the rotor, (d) a flow path for fluid from the harness through the stationary seal into the base of the rotating chamber held in the rotor, the fluid exiting at the top and out the stationary seal to waste or collecting tubes, and (e) a stroboscopic lamp to permit viewing the separation through an aperture in the centrifuge rotor lid. The anticoagulant used for the collection of blood, conditions, rotor speeds, buffer composition, flow rates, and other details related to the isolation of granulocytes from whole blood and buffy coat are detailed elsewhere (Lionetti *et al.,* 1977).

The results of the first 69 of more than 500 blood separation experiments are summarized in Table 1. They show that greater than 90% of granulocytes in whole blood or buffy coat were harvested. From buffy coat leukocytes 99% of the available granulocytes were obtained from ACD and 97% from CPD anticoagulated blood. Heparin was less satisfactory because of lower yields (80%) and higher red cell contamination (10%). Optimum results were obtained with CPD anticoagulated whole blood. Differential counts gave 96% polymorphonuclear leukocytes and 1–3% mononuclear cells. From CPD anticoagulated whole blood, a polymorphonuclear to red blood cell ratio of 41 was obtained ($\approx$2.5% red cells). Properties of granulocytes isolated by counterflow centrifugation were characteristic of normal cells in appearance, volume, oxygen consumption, nucleotide content, chemotaxis, and particle ingestion (Lionetti et al., 1977). Ninety-nine percent of granulocytes produced fluorescein in cytoplasm from fluorescein diacetate and excluded ethidium bromide from their nuclei suggesting high viability of the isolated granulocytes.

Granulocytes of other species have been isolated with similar results. For cryogenic preservation, we have isolated granulocytes from dog, guinea pig (unpublished), and baboon (Lionetti et al., 1978). In other laboratories isolation of granulocytes has been reported in the dog (Jemionek et al., 1978a) and human (Persidsky and Olson, 1978a). Several trials with rat blood were unsuccessful. Despite elevated white cell counts of 20,000 per mm[3], granulocytes of the rat do not separate readily from the mononuclear cells or red cells. About 75% of the white cell count of rats consists of lymphocytes whose diameters are similar to those of red cells. This apparently obviated the separation of the relatively small proportion of granulocytes.

TABLE 1

Isolation of Granulocytes from Whole Blood and Buffy Coat by Counterflow Centrifugation Blood Collected in ACD, CPD, or Heparin [a,b]

Anticoagulant	Number of experiments	Recovery (% of PMNG)	WC Differential count (%)			PMNG	Fluorescence (%)	
			Polys	Lymphs	Other	RBC	Green	Red
Heparin	6	80 ± 15	99.0 ± 0.6	0.5 ± 0.6	0.8 ± 0.8	10	98.6 ± 1.5	1.0 ± 0.0
ACD (% v/v)[c]								
25	21	92 ± 12	97.4 ± 2.1	0.8 ± 0.7	1.8 ± 2.2	4.6	98.6 ± 1.3	1.5 ± 1.3
22	14	91 ± 11	96.4 ± 2.1	1.4 ± 1.1	2.2 ± 1.5	6.9	98.4 ± 0.7	1.6 ± 0.7
15	3	88 ± 7	96.9 ± 1.7	1.8 ± 1.9	1.7 ± 0.3	7.2	98.7 ± 0.3	1.3 ± 0.3
7.5	9	90 ± 8	96.8 ± 2.6	1.2 ± 1.2	1.8 ± 1.5	11	98.2 ± 0.5	2.0 ± 0.7
CPD	6	99 ± 3	98.8 ± 0.4	0.5 ± 0.3	0.7 ± 0.3	24	98.3 ± 0.5	1.7 ± 0.5
Overall	59	91 ± 11	97.3 ± 2.1	1.0 ± 0.9	1.7 ± 1.7	8.8	98.5 ± 0.9	1.5 ± 0.9
ACD (Buffy coat)	6	99 ± 3	95.3 ± 2.9	3.2 1.8	1.3 ± 1.0	17	98.5 ± 0.6	1.5 ± 0.6
CPD (Buffy coat)	4	97 ± 4	96.0 ± 2.0	2.3 1.9	1.8 0.5	41	98.5 ± 0.6	1.5 ± 0.6

[a] All values are means ± s.d.
[b] Reprinted with permission of Transfusion.
[c] ACD, 15% = normal volume concentration.

In the above studies, the granulocytes were pelleted in the chamber by stopping the pump and rotor simultaneously which arrested buffer flow and increased the sedimentation force on the granulocytes. The chamber was then removed and the granulocytes aspirated with a syringe and blunted needle. Other investigators (Nunn and Gagne, 1978; Jemionek *et al.*, 1978a; Persidsky and Olson, 1978) have introduced modifications which permit collection of greater numbers of granulocytes from the rotor without dismantling it. The use of mixing chambers allows for larger volumes of blood to be processed over a longer period with a reduction of purity and recovery of granulocytes (Jemionek *et al.*, 1978a). The replacement of a component of the stationary rotary seal on top of the rotor with a rubber septum allows the insertion of a syringe needle directly into the flow line permitting aspiration of granulocytes. This eliminates the necessity of removing the chamber from the rotor and allows the removal of granulocytes without pelleting them. Repeated runs can then be made without dismantling the rotor (Nunn and Gagne, 1978). Similarly, granulocytes have been flushed from the rotor by means of a reverse-flow valve (Persidsky and Olson, 1978). For the studies published, the numbers of granulocytes isolated have been 1×10^8 to 5×10^8 occupying 0.1–0.5 ml of packed cell volume. Multiple centrifugations have been required to achieve greater yields. Three or four sequential runs taking about 4–5 h is a practical technical period without influencing the stability of isolated granulocytes provided pump speeds and G forces are optimum, and the granulocytes are protected with albumin at temperatures between 4–10°C.

Isolation and preservation of granulocytes of dog and man has been investigated by French, Jemionek, Contreras, Hartwig, and Shields and their manuscripts accepted for publication have been kindly provided to us. These investigators have combined leukopheresis and centrifugal elutriation to fill a 4.5 ml Beckman chamber with approximately 1×10^9 granulocytes. When only counterflow centrifugation was used, high recovery of granulocytes was obtained by starting with 120 ml buffy coat white cell concentrates from canine or human blood and diluting the red cell count to 3×10^8 per ml before transfer to the rotor. From dog blood, 82% of granulocytes were recovered, 96% of which were polymorphonuclear and 4% were mononuclear (Jemionek *et al.*, 1978a). Similarly, 77% of available granulocytes, equal to 3.0×10^8 cells, were recovered from human buffy coat—97% of them were polymorphonuclear and 4% were mononuclear cells (Jemionek *et al.*, 1979). In both studies granulocytes were free of platelets and erythrocytes. *In vitro* tests of chemotactic response, stimulated oxygen consumption, bactericidal capacity, enzyme activities, morphology, and cell volume were performed. No loss of function or morphological integrity due to isolation was observed. When counterflow centrifugation elutriation was combined with leukopheresis by continuous flow centrifugation, maximal use of the Beckman rotor was realized (Contreras *et al.*, 1979). From an average leukopheretic collection containing approximately 5×10^9 human granulocytes, four sequential counterflow centrifugations produced per run 1.4×10^9 granulocytes which was a recovery of 82% of the available granulocytes. The maximum capacity of the elutriation chamber was found to be 1.3×10^9 leukocytes which consisted of 99% granulocytes. The red cell contamination was 2%. The counterflow system used in conjunction with centrifugation was designed for continuous use and collected $4-5 \times 10^9$ granulocytes in 4–5 h with a purity of 95%. The advantage of combining counterflow centrifugation with leukopheresis is the attainability of stable granulocytes at the 1×10^9 magnitude with a high degree of purity, but at a cost of considerable additional time.

III. ISOLATION OF MONOCYTES OF HUMAN BLOOD

Mononuclear cells of human blood are commonly obtained by centrifugation on gradients of albumin (Bennett and Cohn, 1966), sucrose (Zeya *et al.*, 1978), or Ficoll–Isopaque (Loos *et al.*, 1976a), the last being the most widely used method. The adhesiveness of monocytes is used to separate them from lymphocytes in the mixed mononuclear population isolated with the gradient. Monocytes adhere to surfaces of culture flasks (Ackerman and Douglas, 1978; Bennett and Cohn, 1966) or beads (Rabinowitz, 1964), allowing lymphocytes to be washed free. Monocytes are slightly less dense than lymphocytes and centrifugation of Ficoll–Hypaque isolated mononuclear cells on gradients of intermediate specific gravity can be used to separate the two populations. Loos *et al.* (1976a) have isolated monocytes from whole blood using precisely defined discontinuous Ficoll–Isopaque gradients. In all of the procedures devised to date, it has been difficult to obtain pure monocytes in suspension to exceed 50×10^6 cells.

The counterflow elutriation principle has been applied to the isolation of mononuclear cells of human blood in several ways. Lymphocytes, monocytes, and granulocytes were isolated in the Beckman JE-6 rotor in order to study cholesterol biosynthesis (Fogelman *et al.*, 1977). Heparinized whole blood was treated with gelatin to rouleaux and sediment red cells and the white cell rich supernatant plasma removed and separated in the rotor. After loading the chamber, during which residual red cells and platelets were removed, the flow of buffer was increased from 7.8 ml/min to 19 ml/min in increments of 3–4 ml/min every 10 min. Lymphocytes, monocytes, and granulocytes were separated and collected sequentially. Lymphocytes and granulocytes obtained were relatively pure, whereas monocytes were concentrated to 33% purity.

Monocytes with an average purity of 90% were isolated from 10-ml samples of heparinized whole blood from each of six donors by Sanderson and Bird (1977). Mononuclear cells initially isolated on Ficoll–Hypaque gradients were separated by counterflow centrifugation in the Beckman JE-6 rotor in a specially modified chamber (Sanderson *et al.*, 1976). Volume analysis revealed a bimodal monocyte population. Greater than 60% of these were in the large peak (370 μm^3) while the smaller one of 330 μm^3 overlapped the lymphocyte distribution.

Partial resolution of human blood lymphocytes into T and B cells was reported by Griffith (1978) using counterflow centrifugation of the mononuclear cell fraction that was collected with Ficoll–Hypaque. The mononuclear cells from 25 ml of heparinized whole blood were admitted to the chamber of the Beckman rotor and B and T lymphocytes separated at constant G force with three sequential 50 ml changes of buffered bovine albumin varying in concentration from 15 to 21% and in density from 1.011 to 1.019. Four fractions were collected and from the exit port of the chamber five minutes after entry of the 15%, 17%, 19%, and 21% albumin. By means of rosetting techniques for T and B cells, it was found that lymphocytes obtained with 15% albumin were 98% T cells. The collection with 17% albumin contained no cells. In 19% albumin 96% B lymphocytes were obtained. The final increase, to 21% albumin, yielded only cell clumps and granulocytes. The separation of B and T lymphocytes from whole blood probably represents the maximum sensitivity of the Beckman system as presently used.

By adsorption of granulocytes and monocytes on columns of nylon fibers during filtration adhesion leukopheresis and selective elution of granulocytes, Djerassi and associates (1973) found 3–5 × 10^9 mononuclear cells in 100 × 10^9 cells prepared with this procedure. The monocyte fraction was centrifuged on a Ficoll–Hypaque gradient to remove contaminating granulocytes. A mononuclear population containing 75% monocytes was obtained. Where filtration adhesion leukopheresis is used to obtain granulocytes, billions of monocytes are readily available.

A. Isolation of Monocytes by Incremental Flow Elutriation

A superior method for the isolation of large numbers of pure monocytes utilizes incremental flow centrifugal elutriation. The starting material is whole blood or the cells obtained after plateletpheresis, a method for obtaining platelets for clinical transfusion from a single donor by passing the blood through an extra corporeal system to isolate platelet-rich plasma and returning the remainder to the donor. Using the Haemonetics Model 30 Blood Processor, the platelet-rich plasma contains as many as 5×10^9 monocytes that can be concentrated by centrifugation.

Data obtained in this laboratory on the isolation of monocytes from whole blood are shown in Fig. 4 and Table 2. One hundred milliliters of whole blood anticoagulated with CPD was centrifuged to obtain a buffy coat and to remove most of the platelets and plasma. The buffy coats plus packed red cells in a 30-ml volume were diluted threefold with 50% plasma in isotonic sodium chloride and a 35-ml volume was centrifuged in the presence of a Ficoll–Isopaque gradient. Monocytes were then separated from lymphocytes and other contaminating cells by counterflow centrifugation in the Beckman JE-6 rotor by adjusting the flow rates of buffer incrementally at specific time intervals. Figure 4 shows the volume distributions of

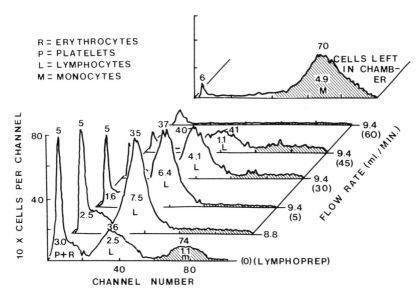

FIGURE 4. Isolation of monocytes from Lymphoprep-separated mononuclear cells of whole blood. A composite of volume distributions is shown for mononuclear cells separated at different flow rates of buffer through the rotor. The initial plot (0) represents the numbers and cell types as cells per channel versus channel number (proportional to size) from Lymphoprep-treated whole blood. The numbers on each peak define the median channel number (midrange) while the numbers under each defines the numbers of cells in the aliquot (0.1 ml) of the population. Successive plots are shown at 5, 30, 45, and 60 min after initiation of the 9.4 ml/min flow rate. The numbers in parenthesis under the flow rates are the times at which the effluent was sampled. The shaded area represents monocytes (M) initially present (time 0), in the elutriations, and remaining in the chamber. The peak at median number 5 in the unshaded area represents platelets and red cells (P + R), peaks at 35–40 represent lymphocytes (L).

TABLE 2
Isolation of Monocytes from Whole Blood[a]

Sample (n = 5)	Total leukocytes (× 10^6)	Myeloperoxidase positive cells (%)	Differential count (% of 200 cells)			Total monocytes × 10^6c	Recovery of monocytes (%)	Microfluorescence (%)[d]		Median channel[e] (no.)
			PMN[b]	Mononuclear	Other			FDA	EB	
Whole blood	555 ± 17 (531–580)	60 ± 5 (53–66)	61 ± 3 (57–65)	37 ± 4 (33–42)	1 ± 1 (0–2)	127 ± 4 (123–132)	—	99 ± 1 (99–100)	1 ± 1 (0–1)	—
Buffy coat	356 ± 59 (272–440)	57 ± 5 (49–64)	64 ± 4 (60–70)	34 ± 4 (30–39)	1 ± 1 (0–1)	69 ± 12 (52–86)	65 ± 15 (42–65)	99 ± 1 (99–100)	1 ± 1 (0–1)	—
Ficoll–Isopaque separated	106 ± 26 (77–130)	28 ± 16 (2–46)	1 ± 1 (0–2)	99 ± 1 (98–99)	0 ± 1 (0–1)	33 ± 16 (16–58)	42 ± 13 (35–42)	98 ± 1 (97–99)	2 ± 1 (1–3)	70 ± 3 (65–75)
Elutriated monos	30 ± 9 (21–45)	93 ± 5 (90–97)	0 ± 1 (0–2)	99 ± 1 (98–99)	1 ± 1 (0–1)	25 ± 9 (16–29)	89 ± 12 (50–100)	98 ± 1 (97–99)	2 ± 1 (1–3)	71 ± 3 (68–74)

[a]The mean ± standard error and the range (parentheses) of each value is reported.
[b]PMN, polymorphonuclear granulocytes.
[c]The total monocytes are calculated as follows: (total leukocytes × % myeloperoxidase positive cells) − (% PMN × myeloperoxidase positive cells).
[d]FDA and EB are the percentages of monocytes that fluoresce with fluorescein diacetate and ethidium bromide.
[e]Median channel is the number representing the midrange in the volume distribution.

cells that were elutriated by sequential increases of flow rate of buffer through the rotor. The volume distributions revealed three populations of cells in the Lymphoprep-treated buffy coat at zero time. The peak with a midrange of 5 corresponds to platelets and red cells. The number 3.0 inside the distribution represents the number of cells (in thousands) in the aliquots counted from Lymphoprep-treated buffy coat. The middle peak marked L refers to lymphocytes (midrange 36) and the large cells in the shaded area marked M are monocytes (midrange 75). Volume distributions are plotted for separations observed when flow rate of buffer through the rotor ranged from 8.8 to 9.4 ml/min. At the 8.8 ml/min rate, large numbers of lymphocytes and contaminant red cells and platelets (nonshaded area) exited from the rotor accompanied by small numbers of monocytes (shaded area). Increase of the flow rate to 9.4 ml/min for 55 min caused all lymphocytes and other cell types to exit with a small loss of monocytes. The volume distribution of cells remaining in the chamber was primarily that of monocytes. The small peak at channel number 6 consisted of cell fragments and red cells. The shoulder to the left of the monocyte peak indicated the presence of less than 1% lymphocytes of several sizes.

Table 2 gives recovery data and some characteristics of monocytes from five experiments. From whole blood 65% of available monocytes were found in buffy coat and 42% of these were isolated with Ficoll–Isopaque. Of these 89% were recovered in the chamber of the rotor after counterflow centrifugation and elutriation of the other cell types. The differential white blood cell counts of Wright-stained smears revealed 99% of the cells were monocytes with a few polymorphonuclear cells and red cells. Ninety-eight percent of the cells reacted positively with fluorescein diacetate and 2% reacted with ethidium bromide. These findings indicate that monocytes had viable cytoplasmic and nuclear membranes. At the suggestion of R. Yankee, we have scaled our techniques to use plateletpheresis cell residues and have isolated and successfully preserved by cryogenic methods 1 to 5 $\times$ 10^9 homogeneous monocytes (Hunt *et al.*, 1980).

IV. APPRAISAL OF COUNTERFLOW CENTRIFUGATION FOR THE ISOLATION OF LEUKOCYTES

A. Who Needs 1 × 10^8 Granulocytes?

From the foregoing it is apparent that counterflow centrifugation elutriation is a useful method for the isolation of specific white cell types ordinarily difficult because of small numbers or differences in size and density. The Beckman JE-6 rotor and elutriation system can separate 1 $\times$ 10^8 granulocytes in one step from 25 ml of whole blood (see Table 1). The elutriated granulocytes have normal morphological, biochemical, and physiological functions. A distinct advantage is that the separation of granulocytes, one of the most unstable of the cell types in blood, takes place in media ideal with respect to composition, pH, and molarity for their optimum stability. The counterflow of buffer results in net G forces significantly less than simple centrifugation. Of high value is the purity of granulocytes isolated, particularly the absence of mononuclear cells and the low red cell contamination.

The granulocytes obtained by the counterflow centrifugation method can be used for typing antigens, to detect granulocyte cytotoxic antibodies, to study granulocyte circulation and distribution to tissue, and to study methods of preservation. Our studies on liquid (Contreras *et al.,* 1978a) and cryogenic (Lionetti *et al.,* 1978) preservation have been facilitated by the freedom from contaminant cells. The absence of platelets renders granulocytes stable at 4°C for days and the absence of mononuclear cells makes unequivocal the elucidation of properties unique to granulocytes.

The isolation of mononuclear cells of blood by the counterflow centrifugation method is now possible and this technology must now be evaluated with centrifugal, immunological, or electronic cell-sorting methods. However, by means of stepwise or sequential changes in flow rates and elutriation media, the separation of many biological cell types have been reported and recently reviewed (Pretlow and Pretlow, 1979). By incremental increases in flow rates Fogelman *et al.* (1977) separated and collected lymphocytes, monocytes, and granulocytes from one sedimented whole blood sample. Similarly, we have isolated monocytes from Ficoll–Isopaque treated buffy coat leukocytes.

B. Scaling the Numbers to 1×10^{10} Granulocytes

Leukopheretic methods of white cell collection provide granulocytes of the 1×10^{10} magnitude (Huestis, 1977). Leukopheresis, using centrifugal methods, yields mixtures of all blood cells similar in composition to buffy coat cells obtained by simple centrifugation. In these, the granulocytes are greatly outnumbered by platelets and red cells and contain mononuclear cells of approximately equal magnitude. Although clinically useful, the need remains to isolate therapeutically required numbers of homogeneous granulocytes. Technology does not exist presently which can do it. (Methods to collect granulocytes by leukopheresis will be described elsewhere in this book.)

Counterflow centrifugation elutriation has been employed following leukopheresis to concentrate granulocytes and remove contaminant cells in dog (Jemionek *et al.*, 1978b) and human (Contreras *et al.*, 1979). These authors demonstrated that 5×10^9 homogeneous granulocytes with high *in vitro* function could be isolated in multiple elutriations. This procedure requires at least a half day to complete. The value for clinical transfusion purposes is thus compromised by the inadequacy of numbers, the time required, and the complexity of the procedure.

The counterflow elutriation principle is employed in the Cell Separator 3000 (Fenwal) scaled for the sterile collection in plastic bags of 1×10^{10} granulocytes in about 2 h. From whole blood of a donor with an average granulocyte count of 38,000 per mm^3, it is claimed that 75% can be isolated with a differential white blood cell count of 80% granulocytes and 20% mononuclear cells. Platelets are approximately equal to granulocytes and red cells 3–5 times as much. Instruments like this hold promise that granulocytes in numbers required for clinical transfusion are obtainable with significant reduction, although not the elimination of platelets, red cells, and mononuclear cells.

The combined techniques of plateletpheresis or leukopheresis with counterflow centrifugation elutriation currently makes feasible the isolation of 1 to 10×10^9 monocytes to 1 to 10×10^{10} granulocytes. Although technically difficult, the advantage of homogeneity and freedom from other cell types may justify limited utility of the combined techniques. For experimental purposes counterflow centrifugation elutriation is well suited to the separation of stem cells or colony-forming activity in whole blood or bone marrow where the mononuclear cells in the fractions isolated are of the order of 1 to 10×10^8 in number.

C. Some Technical Considerations

The technical requirements for use of counterflow centrifugation procedure require an hour to set up the hardware and software, up to 2 h to operate when stepwise flow rates are utilized, and a half-hour to clean up after the procedure. A disadvantage is that the Beckman rotor must be disassembled daily to be cleaned and sterilized. The various components, including rings, springs, bushing, and harness, must be cleaned after use. After assembly, the rotor, tubing, and accessories are flushed daily with 100 ml of 10% Chlorox and then flushed with 1 liter of sterile phosphate-buffered saline. Cultures of the effluent are negative when the rotor and accessories are properly cleaned. In addition, prior to use, the system must be purged of air.

The stroboscopic lamp is synchronized and aligned with a hole in the rotor and centrifuge cover so that the chamber can be visualized during the addition of blood or cell suspensions and the separation within the chamber can be visualized. The color of the blood in the chamber is initially red and as the separation occurs, the red cells leave and the color changes progressively to white. The cell–buffer interface can be observed and the separation modified with small adjustments of the flow rate. The separation is completed when only the grey-white granulocytes remain. Occasionally, small clumps of cells are visible which tend to remain in the chamber and are aspirated as contaminants with granulocytes. To minimize contaminant clumps, granulocytes can be removed while the rotor is running by reverse flushing or by aspiration of the granulocytes using a needle inserted into the septum. We have minimized clumping by removal of platelets from the cell product that is placed into the chamber and by silicone coating of the chamber.

We have found that identification of the leukocytes and the quantitation of cell recovery by stained smears to be time-consuming. Instead we have utilized the volume distribution of cells and microfluorescent measurements to test the isolated cells. The size of the cells and number of cells within each distribution can be used to assess the purity and stability of the cell population. Other investigators have likewise utilized volume distributions to characterize monocytes (Sanderson *et al.*, 1977) and monocytes and lymphocytes (Loos *et al.*, 1976b). We used microfluorescence measurements to measure cytoplasmic and nuclear membrane integrity and serum dependent latex and yeast ingestion to assess phagocytic function. These tests require only 1×10^5 cells and are simple to perform.

REFERENCES

Ackerman, S. K., and Douglas, S. D., 1978, Purification of human monocytes on microexudate-coated surfaces, *J. Immunol* **120**:1372.
Bennett, W. E., and Cohn, Z. A. 1966, The isolation and selected properties of blood monocytes, *J. Exp. Med.* **123**:145.
Contreras, T. J., Hunt, S. M., Lionetti, F. J., and Valeri, C. R., 1978a, Preservation of human granulocytes. III. Liquid preservation studied by electronic sizing, *Transfusion* **18**:46.
Contreras, T. J., Jemionek, J. F., French, J. E., and Hartwig, V., 1978b, Liquid preservation of canine granulocytes obtained by counterflow centrifugation, *Exp. Hematol. (Copenhagen)* **6**:767.
Contreras, T. J., Jemionek, J. F., French, F. E., and Shields, L. J., 1979, Human granulocyte isolation by continuous flow centrifugation leukopheresis and counterflow centrifugation-elutriation, *Transfusion* (in press).
Djerassi, I., Kim, J. S., and Suvansri, U., 1973, Harvesting human monocytes as a by-product of filtration-leukophoresis, *Proc. Am. Assoc. Cancer Res.* **14**:103 (Abstr.).
Fogelman, A. M., Seager, J., Edwards, P. A. Kokom, M., and Popjak, G., 1977, Cholesterol biosynthesis in human lymphocytes, monocytes and granulocytes, *Biochem. Biophys. Res. Commun.* **76**:167.
Grabske, R. J., 1978, Separating cell populations by elutriation. Fractions, *Beckman Bull.* **1**:1.

Griffith, O. M., 1978, Separation of human T and B cells from human peripheral blood by centrifugal elutriation, *Anal. Biochem.* **87**:97.

Huestis, D. W., 1977, Production, storage and histocompatibility of granulocytes, in *Blood Leukocytes Functions and Use in Therapy* C. H. Hogman, K. Lindahl-Kiessling, and H. Higzell, eds.), Reklam and Katalogtryk, Uppsala, p. 55.

Hunt, S. M., Lionett, F. J., and Valeri, C. R., 1980, Isolation and cryogenic preservation of human blood monocytes (in preparation).

Jemionek, J. F., Contreras, T. J., Frenceh, J. E., and Hartwig, V., 1978a, Improved technique for increased granulocyte recovery from canine whole blood samples by counterflow centrifugation elutriation. I. *In vitro* analysis, *Exp. Hematol. (Copenhagen)* **6**:558.

Jemionek, J. F., Contreras, T. J., French, J. F., and Shields, L. J., 1978b, Granulocyte isolation by counterflow centrifugation elutriation of canine blood obtained by continuous flow centrifugation leukopheresis, *Exp. Hematol. (Copenhagen)* **6**:801.

Jemionek, J. F., Contreras, T. C., French, J. E., and Shields, L. J., 1979, Technique for increased granulocyte recovery from human whole blood by counterflow centrifugation elutriation. I. *In vitro* analysis, *Transfusion* **19**:120.

Lindahl, P. E., 1948, Principle of a counterstreaming centrifuge for the separation of particles of different sizes, *Nature* **161**:648.

Lindahl, P. E., and Lindahl, K. M., 1955, On the concentration of eosinophile leukocytes, *Experientia* **11**:310.

Lindahl, P. E., 1956, On counterstreaming centrifugation in the separation of cells and cell fragments, *Biochim. Biophys. Acta* **21**:411.

Lionetti, F. J., Hunt, S. M., Lin, P. S., Kurtz, S. R., and Valeri, C. R., 1977, Preservation of human granulocytes. II. Characteristics of granulocytes obtained by counterflow centrifugation, *Transfusion* **17**:465.

Lionetti, F. J., Hunt, S. M., Mattaliano, R. J., and Valeri, C. R., 1978, *In vitro* studies of cryopreserved baboon granulocytes, *Transfusion* **18**:685.

Loos, H., Blok-Schut, B., Van Doorn, R., Hoksbergen, R., and Brutel de la Riviere, A., 1976a, A method for the recognition and separation of human blood monocytes on density gradients, *Blood* **48**:731.

Loos, H., Blok-Schut, B., Kipp, B., Van Doorn, R., and Meerhof, L., 1976b, Size distribution, electronic recognition and counting of human blood monocytes, *Blood* **48**:720.

McEwen, C. R., Stallard, R. W. and Juhos, and E. Th.,1968, Separation of biological particles by centrifugal elutriations, *Anal. Biochem.* **23**:369.

McEwen, C. R., Juhos, E. Th., Stallard, R. W., Schnell, J. V., Siddiqui, W. A., and Geiman, Q. M., 1971, Centrifugal elutriation for the removal of leukocytes from malaria-infected monkey blood, *J. Parasitol.* **57**:887.

Nunn, A. D., and Gagne, G., 1978, The recovery in small volume of cells from the Beckman JE-6 rotor, *Transfusion* **18**:599.

Persidsky, M. D., and Olson, L. S., 1978, Granulocyte separation by modified centrifugal elutriation system, *Proc. Soc. Exp. Biol. Med.* **157**:599.

Pretlow, T. G., and Pretlow, T. P., 1979, Centrifugal elutriation (counterstreaming centrifugation) of cells, *Cell Biophys.* **1**:195.

Rabinowitz, Y., 1964, Separation of lymphocytes, polymorphonuclear leukocytes and monocytes on glass columns, including tissue culture observations, *Blood* **23**:811.

Sanderson, R. J., and Bird, K. E., 1977, Cell separation by counterflow centrifugation, in *Methods in Cell Biology* (D. M. Prescott, ed.), pp. 1–14, Academic Press, New York.

Sanderson R. J., Bird, K. E., Palmer, N. F., and Brenman, J., 1976, Design principles for counterflow centrifugation cell separation chamber, *Anal. Biochem.* **71**:615.

Sanderson, R. J., Sheppardson, F. T., Valter, A. E., and Talmadge, D. W., 1977, Isolation and enumeration of peripheral blood monocytes, *J. Immunol.* **118**:1409.

Zeya, H. I. Keku, E., De Chatelet, L. R., Cooper, M. R., and Spurr, C. L., 1978, Isolation of enzymatically homogeneous populations of human leukocytes, monocytes and granulocytes by zonal centrifugation, *Am. J. Pathol.* **90**:33.

Biological Methods for the Separation of Lymphoid Cells

CHRIS D. PLATSOUCAS AND NICHOLAS CATSIMPOOLAS

I. GENERAL CONSIDERATIONS

Presently, it has been conclusively established that three major classes of cells are involved in the immune response (Miller and Mitchell, 1969; Katz and Benacerraf, 1972; Good, 1972): T lymphocytes which are thymus-dependent and responsible for the so-called cell-mediated immunity and overall regulation of the immune response; B lymphocytes which are thymus independent and functional in the humoral aspects of immunity; and macrophages (and monocytes) which "process" and present the antigen to T lymphocytes and, therefore, regulate the immune response by rather nonspecific means. These three major classes of lymphoid cells, and especially the T and B lymphocytes, are further subdivided to a large number of functionally distinct subpopulations (Stout and Herzenberg, 1975; Lobo *et al.*, 1975; Murphy *et al.*, 1976; Scher *et al.*, 1976; Press *et al.*, 1976; Cantor and Boyse, 1976; Moretta *et al.*, 1977), so that the overall picture of the individual cell types forming the lymphoid cell system appears very complex. The significance and need for cell separation methods in studies of this complex system is obvious. Experiments designed to identify the functional role of lymphocyte subpopulations require "homogeneous" or "pure" populations of cells. Furthermore, precise functional and structural characterization of cells from lymphoproliferative and myeloproliferative

CHRIS D. PLATSOUCAS AND NICHOLAS CATSIMPOOLAS • Biophysics Laboratory, Department of Nutrition and Food Science, Massachusetts Institute of Technology, Cambridge, Massachusetts 02139. Present Address for CDP: Memorial Sloan-Kettering Cancer Center, New York, New York 10021.

disorders can be accomplished only with relatively homogeneous abnormal cell populations. Transfusion, bone marrow transplantation (prevention of the graft-vs-host disease), and immunotherapy are some of the other areas where sophisticated cell separation methods are required. Another field of active research where cell separation methods are urgently required is cell hybridization. The production of hybridomas exhibiting specific biological functions is greatly facilitated if functionally distinct lymphocyte populations of high purity are available as starting material. In addition, the availability of the latter simplifies the difficult and tedious problem of selection of the cell hybrids.

Available methods for separation of lymphoid cells are generally divided into two categories, those based on physical properties and those which depend on biological characteristics (Häyry et al., 1975). Although a combination of biological and physical methods is what is actually used in the immunological laboratory, the above general methodological classification is certainly valid. The biological methods take advantage of specific biological or functional characteristics of cells selectively expressed on distinct subpopulations. The physical methods utilize differences in physical properties of cells such as size, density, cell surface charge, etc., to achieve separation. Based on one or more of these physical properties, the following methods for the separation of lymphoid cells have been employed: (1) sedimentation velocity, (2) buoyant density centrifugation, (3) electrophoresis, (4) physical adherence, (5) countercurrent distribution, and (6) cell sorting. All of the above methods have been examined in detail in these series and will not be discussed here.

The majority of the biological methods of cell separation are based on the presence of different receptors or cell surface antigens, selectively expressed on certain lymphocyte populations. These are clonal or class receptors (e.g., immunoglobulins), differentiation, or histocompatibility antigens, and either involve or mediate specific immunological functions such as antigen recognition and regulation of the immune response, recognition of altered-self, and cell-mediated cytolysis, or they are products of differentiation pathways with unknown immunological function (e.g., Ly antigens). The most commonly employed receptors in cell separation methods are given in Tables 1 and 2, for human and mouse lymphocytes (and monocytes), respectively. Additional biological methods are based on acquired proliferative or metabolic properties of cells, or cell surface receptors for lectins.

The following biological methods for separation of lymphoid cells have been described in the literature:

1. Rosetting
2. Cellular immunoabsorbents; affinity chromatography

TABLE 1
Receptors or Markers on Human Lymphocytes and Monocytes

Receptor or marker	Cell population		
	T	B	Monocytes
E[a]	+	−	−
Fc(IgG)[b]	Tγ only	+	+
Fc (IgM)[c]	Tμ only	+	?
CR I(b)[d]	−	+	+
CR II(d)[e]	−	+	+
EBV[f]	−	+	−
MRBC[g]	−	+	−
SIg[h]	−	+	−

[a]E, receptor for sheep red blood cells.
[b]Fc, receptor for IgG.
[c]Fc, receptor for IgM.
[d]Complement receptor I or b.
[e]Complement receptor II or d.
[f]Receptor for Epstein–Barr virus.
[g]Receptor for mouse red blood cells.
[h]Surface immunoglobulin, mainly IgDκ and IgMκ.

3. Negative selection (elimination) by treatment of the cells with an antiserum to a surface antigen and complement
4. "Suicide" of a proliferating cell population by incorporation of radioactive isotope of high specific activity
5. Methods based on the reversible binding of lectins on certain lymphocyte subpopulations, bearing the appropriate receptors

TABLE 2
Receptors or Markers on Mouse Lymphocytes and Macrophages

Receptor or marker	Cell population		
	T	B	Macrophages
Theta-antigen	+	−	−
Ly-1	T-helper	−	−
Ly-23	T-suppressor	−	−
Fc[a]	Few	+	+
CR I(b)[b]	−	+	+
CR II(d)[c]	−	+	−
SIg[d], mainly IgM and IgD	−	+	−

[a]Fc receptor for IgG.
[b]Complement receptor I or b.
[c]Complement receptor II or d.
[d]Surface immunoglobulin.

The text that follows gives an overview of biological methods for lymphoid cell separation with the aim to provide an operational guide rather than to describe methodological details. The discussion will be essentially limited to preparative techniques. Methods dealing only with the detection or enumeration of lymphoid cell subpopulations will not be presented.

II. ROSETTING METHODS

A. Introduction

Lymphocytes from several species upon reaction with heterologous (or autologous) native or specific antibody-coated erythrocytes form structures known as rosettes where a single lymphocyte is surrounded by a number of attached erythrocytes. Presumably any molecule that can react with a lymphocyte surface antigen (or it can bind to a lymphocyte surface receptor)—if attached to the surface of erythrocytes—may lead to rosette formation. In addition, lymphocytes from several species have receptors for certain native heterologous erythrocytes (e.g., sheep, mouse, monkey). Rosette formation of functionally distinct lymphocyte subpopulations is usually an easy and convenient method for the quantitative determination of these cells. Furthermore, rosetting is frequently used for the preparative separation of cells by taking advantage of differences in the physical properties (density and size) between the rosettes and the remaining nonrosetting lymphocytes.

B. Spontaneous Rosettes of Sheep Erythrocytes with Human T Lymphocytes

The formation of spontaneous rosettes between unsensitized sheep erythrocytes (SRBC) and nonimmune human lymphocytes was independently described by a number of investigators (Bach et al., 1969; Brain et al., 1970; Coombs et al., 1970; Lay et al., 1971). Subsequent studies clearly established spontaneous SRBC rosettes as a human T lymphocyte marker (Coombs et al., 1970; Wybran and Fudenberg, 1971; Frøland, 1972; Jondal et al., 1972; Wybran et al., 1972). B lymphocytes and nonlymphoid cells [with the possible exception of certain granulocytes (Hsu and Fell, 1974)] do not form E rosettes. Almost all human thymocytes form E rosettes (Wybran et al., 1972) larger than those formed by peripheral blood lymphocytes (PBL) and stable at 37°C (Yu, 1975; Galili and Schlesinger, 1975). Approximately 80% of normal peripheral blood lymphocytes form E rosettes, under optimal conditions. However, reports from a number of laboratories provide a wide range (20–80%) of E-rosetting cells. These differences are due to variable experimental procedures. Small variations in pH (Chaves and Arranhado, 1972; Braganza *et al.*, 1975), centrifugation time, sample of SRBC, age of the donor sheep, storage of the cells (Kaplan and Clark, 1974; Steel *et al.*, 1975), mechanical trauma during resuspension, and incubation time and temperature may result in wide variations in the number of rosette-forming cells (Chapel, 1973; Mendes *et al.*, 1973; Gupta and Grieco, 1974; Heier, 1974; Smith *et al.*, 1975; Hoffman and Kunkel, 1976; Jondal, 1976a). The presence of AB human or fetal calf serum enhances the adherence of sheep erythrocytes to the lymphocytes. Both the SRBCs bound per lymphocyte and the number of rosetting lymphocytes are increased (Brain *et al.*, 1970; Bentwich *et al.*, 1973). The absorption of the serum, prior to the assay, with sheep red blood cells is a rather common practice (Hoffman and Kunkel, 1976; Winchester and Ross, 1976). However, this step may not be necessary at least for preselected lots of fetal calf serum (West *et al.*, 1978).

A typical rosetting procedure proceeds as follows. Lymphocytes are mixed with sheep erythrocytes at a ratio in the range of 20–100 erythrocytes per lymphocyte and the mixture is centrifuged at $50g$ or $100g$ for 5 min, thus providing maximum lymphocyte–RBC contact. The rosettes are enumerated and reported immediately as "short-incubation" or "early rosettes" (Yu, 1975), after incubation at 29°C for 1–18 h as "high-affinity" E rosettes (West *et al.*, 1977b), or after incubation at 4°C overnight as "total rosettes." Incubation at 4°C is required for the detection of all the E-rosette-forming cells. A lymphocyte with three or more attached SRBC is considered as a rosette-forming cell and counted as positive. Dead cells and monocytes are excluded from counting. Incubation of the lymphocyte–SRBC mixture for 5 min at 37°C prior to centrifugation increases rosette stability. However, already centrifuged E rosettes from PBL disintegrate after incubation at 37°C (Jondal *et al.*, 1972; Mendes *et al.*, 1973; Steel *et al.*, 1975) in contrast to rosettes formed by thymocytes. Rosettes formed after preincubation of lymphocytes at 37°C for 1 h in high concentration of fetal calf serum, followed by addition of the SRBC, centrifugation, and immediate resuspension at room temperature, are known as "active rosettes" (Wybran and Fudenberg, 1973). Only a 25% to 35% of human peripheral blood lymphocytes produce "active rosettes." It appears that these are associated with a subpopulation of T lymphocytes which is dramatically decreased in cancer and other diseases (Wybran and Fudenberg, 1973; Wybran *et al.*, 1974; Gross *et al.*, 1975; Florey and Peetoom, 1976; Taniguchi *et al.*, 1976).

A number of modifications aiming to improve the rosette assay and especially to reduce the fragility of the rosettes have been reported in the literature. The most frequently used technique is the treatment of sheep erythrocytes with neuraminidase. This treatment enhances the binding of the latter to human T lymphocytes and reduces significantly the fragility of the rosettes (Weiner *et al.*, 1973). Neuraminidase treated SRBC bind only to T lymphocytes (Gilbertsen and Metzgar, 1976). Neuraminidase removes sialic acid from the surface of the RBC (Uhlenbruck *et al.*, 1967) and, by reducing their net negative surface charge (Seaman and Uhlenbruck, 1963), facilitates binding to the T cells. An alternate method employs sheep red blood cells treated with 2-*S*-aminoethyl-isothiouronium bromide (AET), a sulfhydryl compound. Employing SRBC treated with AET "large, stable and quite resistant to mechanical disruption" rosettes can be obtained in less than an hour incubation time (Kaplan and Clark, 1974; Pellegrino *et al.*, 1976; Kaplan *et al.*, 1976). The mechanism of action of AET is not known. Other reports suggest that addition of dextran (Brown *et al.*, 1975), or papain treatment of SRBC improves the stability of the rosettes (Bach, 1973; Dwyer, 1976).

The high density of the erythrocytes (1.12 g/cm^3) and the large size of the rosette structures permits easy separation of the rosetting from the non-rosetting lymphocytes on the basis of their physical properties (density and size). This separation is accomplished by centrifugation of the rosetting and nonrosetting mixture of cells on Ficoll–Hypaque density cushion [density 1.077 g/cm^3 (Bøyum, 1968)]. The method is described in detail elsewhere (Wahl *et at.*, 1974; Mendes *et al.*, 1974; MacDermott *et al.*, 1975; Greaves and Brown, 1974; Pellegrino *et al.*, 1976; Saxon *et al.*, 1976; Wahl *et al.*, 1976). Neuraminidase- or AET-treated sheep red blood cells are usually used. The cells are layered carefully on top of the Ficoll–Hypaque density cushion and centrifuged for 20–30 min at $400g$ (Fig. 1). Rosettes and free SRBC are collected from the bottom of the cushion. Nonrosetting lympho-cytes remain at the interface and are removed with a Pasteur pipette. Free or lymphocyte-attached sheep red blood cells are removed by hypotonic lysis with Tris or KHCO$_3$-buffered ammonium chloride (Boyle, 1968; Kay *et al.*, 1977). The hypotonic treatment abolishes the antibody-dependent cell-mediated cytotoxicity (ADCC) and natural killer (NK) activity of the cells, but it does not seem to affect other properties (Kay *et al.*, 1977). Both ADCC and NK activity return to normal after culturing the cells for 24 h at room temperature. An alternative way to recover the lymphocytes is dissociation of the rosettes by incubation at 37°C and mechanical disrup-tion. Sheep red blood cells are removed by centrifugation on Ficoll–Hypaque density cushion. A similar method has been reported for the iso-lation of human T lymphocytes from tumor tissues (Jondal, 1976a).

Recently, two subpopulations of E-rosetting lymphocytes were described on the basis of their relative affinity for sheep red blood cells (West *et al.*, 1976; Djeu *et al.*, 1977; West *et al.*, 1977a,b). High-affinity E-

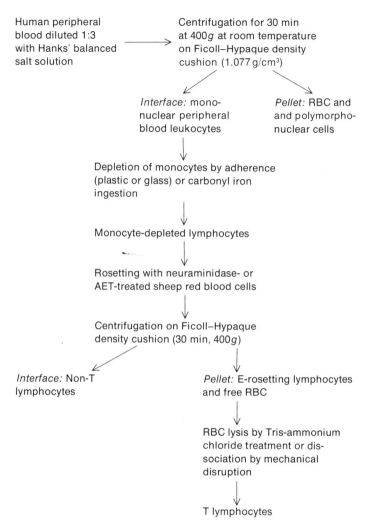

FIGURE 1.   Diagrammatic presentation of T lymphocyte separation by rosetting.

rosette-forming cells can form rosettes with reduced concentrations or SRBC, which are stable after prolonged incubation (1–18 h) at 29°C. These cells account for 54 ± 5% of the mononuclear leukocyte cell fraction (West *et al.*, 1977b). Low-affinity E-rosette-forming cells require considerably higher SRBC concentrations and incubation at 4°C. Low-affinity E rosettes dissociate if incubated at higher temperature. T lymphocytes forming low-

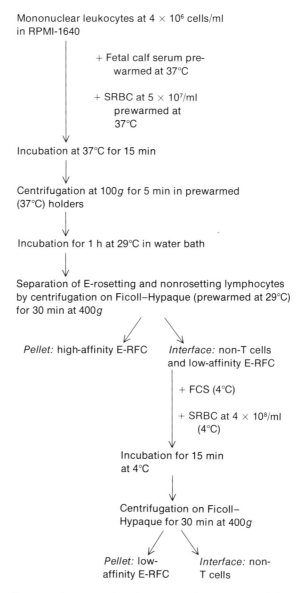

FIGURE 2. Diagrammatic presentation of the preparative separation of high- and low-affinity E-rosette-forming cells (E-RFC) (West *et al.*, 1977b, 1978). For separation of low-affinity E-rosette-forming cells 4 × 10⁸ SRBC/ml were used. The high cell concentration at the Ficoll–Hypaque interface permits rosette formation *in situ*.

affinity E rosettes account for 23 ± 4% of the mononuclear leukocyte cell fraction and include a subpopulation of T cells that are effectors in ADCC (West et al., 1978). Using the appropriate SRBC concentrations and selecting the incubation temperature West et al. (1977a) were able to separate high- and low-affinity E-rosette-forming cells on a preparative scale. This separation procedure is diagrammatically presented in Fig. 2. In another report West et al. (1977b) demonstrated that up to 85% of the low-affinity E-rosette-forming T lymphocytes bear receptors for the Fc portion of IgG whereas only very few (2 ± 1%) of the high-affinity E-rosetting cells had this receptor.

Finally it should be mentioned that human T lymphocytes can be isolated by an indirect rosetting technique, using rabbit anti-human-T-cell serum and sheep erythrocytes coated via $CrCl_3$ (see Section II.F) with anti-rabbit immunoglobulin antibody (Strelkauskas et al., 1975). T lymphocytes coated with rabbit anti-T-cell serum form rosettes with anti-rabbit immunoglobulin antibody-coated SRBC, which subsequently are separated by centrifugation on Ficoll–Hypaque density cushion. T lymphocytes are recovered after lysis of the erythrocytes by Tris-ammonium chloride treatment. This indirect immunocytoadhesion method has also been employed for the separation of JRA-positive from JRA-negative T lymphocytes in humans (Strelkauskas et al., 1978). Peripheral blood T lymphocytes were reacted with sera from patients with juvenile rheumatoid arthritis and rosetted with erythrocytes coated with rabbit anti-human light-chain antibodies. JRA-negative T lymphocytes were separated from JRA-positive cells by centrifugation on Ficoll–Hypaque density cushion. The different functional properties of these human T-cell subsets are described by Strelkauskas et al. (1978).

C. Separation of Human Lymphocyte Subpopulations Bearing Fc Receptors

A large number of lymphoid and myeloid cells in humans and experimental animals bear receptors of variable affinity for the Fc portion of IgG or IgM as summarized in Table 1. These include human T and B lymphocytes (Dickler et al., 1974; Chiao et al., 1974, 1975; Chiao and Good, 1976; Moretta et al., 1975; Ferrarini et al., 1975; Dickler and Kunkel, 1972; Hallberg et al., 1973; Pichler and Knapp, 1978), "third population" cells (Bach et al., 1970; Frøland and Natvig, 1973; Frøland et al., 1974), and T and B lymphocytes from mice and other animal species (Stout and Herzenberg, 1975; Yoshida and Andersson, 1972; VanBoxel and Rosenstreich, 1974; Yodoi et al., 1978). Furthermore, eosinophils, granulocytes (Gupta et al.,

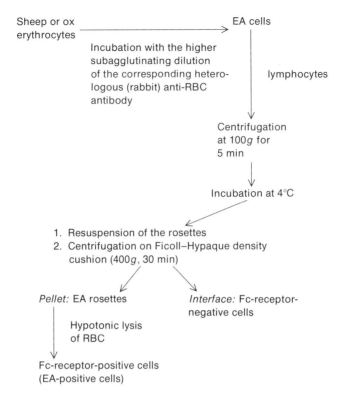

FIGURE 3.   Separation of Fc-receptor-bearing lymphocytes by rosetting methods.

1976b), monocytes (Huber *et al.*, 1969) and certain tumor cells (Tönder *et al.*, 1974) bear Fc receptors.

Rosettes with ox, sheep, or chicken erythrocytes, coated with the appropriate (IgG or IgM) heterologous (rabbit) anti-RBC antibody are used for the detection of cells bearing Fc receptors (Hallberg *et al.*, 1973; Zighelboim *et al.*, 1974; Samarut *et al.*, 1976). Preparative isolation of the Fc-receptor-bearing cells (EA-positive cells) is accomplished by centrifugation on Ficoll–Hypaque density cushion as shown in Fig. 3. In consideration of the expression of Fc receptors by several cell types, separation of the EA-positive cells from heterogeneous cell populations (e.g., peripheral blood mononuclear leukocytes) cannot provide functionally distinct lymphocyte subpopulations. This can be accomplished by separating the Fc-receptor-bearing cells from purified cell populations (e.g., T or B lymphocytes).

1. Separation of Human T Lymphocyte Subpopulations Bearing Receptors for IgM and IgG

Human T lymphocytes have been recently classified into three subpopulations on the basis of the presence of Fc receptors. The $T\mu$ cells have receptors for IgM and represent approximately 55% of the peripheral blood T lymphocytes. The $T\gamma$ cells bear receptors for IgG and account for 10–15% of peripheral blood T cells. The $T\phi$ cells lack receptors for IgM and IgG and account for the remaining proportion of the peripheral blood T cells (Webb and Cooper, 1973; Dickler et al., 1974; Chiao et al., 1974, 1975; Chiao and Good, 1976; Moretta et al., 1975; Ferrarini et al., 1975; Gmelig-Meyling et al., 1976). The $T\mu$ subpopulation contains lymphocytes that exhibit helper activity for the B cell differentiation to immunoglobulin synthesizing and secreting plasma cells, in the pokeweed mitogen-induced system. $T\gamma$ lymphocytes, when activated by immune complexes, contain cells exhibiting suppressor activity in the same system (Moretta et al., 1977). Furthermore, $T\mu$ and $T\gamma$ cells are different in regard to a large number of morphological, structural, and functional properties (Gupta and Good, 1978; Moretta et al., 1978).

$T\mu$ and $T\gamma$ lymphocytes are detected in T-cell-purified populations by rosette formation with ox erythrocytes coated respectively with rabbit IgM or IgG anti-ox-RBC antibodies. The same procedure has been employed for the preparative separation of $T\mu$ and $T\gamma$ cells (Moretta et al., 1976a, 1977; Gupta and Good, 1978; Gupta et al., 1978). The use of ox erythrocytes is obligatory especially for the separation of $T\mu$ cells. Erythrocytes from other species were found unsatisfactory. The separation procedure is presented in Fig. 4. This method of separation of $T\mu$ and $T\gamma$ cells is relatively simple to perform and provides viable and metabolically active lymphocytes. However, it results in modulation of the Fc receptors of the cells with consequent modification of a number of their functional properties (Moretta et al., 1976a; Cordier et al., 1977; Gupta et al., 1978). Recently it has been shown that $T\mu$ and $T\gamma$ cells can be separated by density gradient electrophoresis, without modulation of their Fc receptors (Platsoucas et al., 1979).

2. Separation of Effector Cells (Killer Cells) in Antibody-Dependent Cell-Mediated Cytotoxicity (ADCC) Bearing High-Affinity Receptors for Human IgG

Human erythrocytes (Rh-positive) coated with human anti-Rh serum (Ripley) have been used for the separation of a human peripheral blood

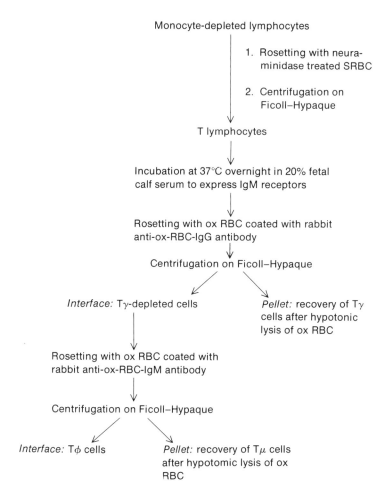

FIGURE 4. Rosetting methods for isolation of $T\mu$, $T\gamma$, and $T\phi$ cells.

lymphocyte subpopulation bearing high-affinity Fc (IgG) receptors (Bach *et al.*, 1970; Frøland and Natvig, 1973; Frøland *et al.*, 1974). Rosetting cells were separated from non-rosetting cells on a Ficoll–Hypaque density cushion as illustrated in Fig. 3. Detailed experimental procedures have been reported elsewhere (Perlmann *et al.*, 1976; Natvig and Frøland, 1976; Frøland and Wisløff, 1976). The isolated cell fractions bearing high-affinity Fc (IgG) receptors are effector cells in antibody-dependent cell-mediated cytotoxicity (ADCC) and in natural killer (NK) cytotoxicity assays. These cells were considered as "third population" cells being non-T, non-B lymphocytes (Frøland and Natvig, 1973; Kurnick and Grey, 1975). However, recent reports suggest that low-affinity E-rosette-forming cells bearing Fc receptor for IgG are also effector cells in ADCC and NK (Kay *et al.*, 1977; Gupta *et al.*, 1978). A fraction of these cells are probably also present in K-cell preparations isolated by this particular rosetting technique.

D. Separation of Lymphocyte Subpopulations Bearing Complement Receptors

A large number of different cell types bear receptors for various complement components including B lymphocytes (Bianco *et al.*, 1970; Bianco and Nussenzweig, 1971; Dierich *et al.*, 1974), "third population" cells in humans (Perlmann *et al.*, 1972), macrophages, monocytes, granulocytes (Ross and Polley, 1975; Griffin *et al.*, 1975; Rabellino and Metcalf, 1975; Ross *et al.*, 1976), eosinophils (Gupta *et al.*, 1976b), and glomerular epithelial cells (Gelfand *et al.*, 1976). Furthermore, up to 2% of the peripheral blood lymphocytes bear receptors for both SRBC and complement (Chiao *et al.*, 1974).

Two distinct complement receptors are reported on mononuclear leukocytes: the immune adherence receptor or CR I or C3b or b receptor and the CR II or d receptor (Ross *et al.*, 1973; Ross and Polley, 1975). These receptors are antigenically distinct and cap independently. The CR I binds to the C3c region of the C3b (fixed on the red blood cell membrane after cleavage of the C3b by the enzyme C3 convertase) and to a similar amino acid sequence on the C4. The CR II receptor binds to the C3d region of the C3b as well as to the C3d region when bound to the erythrocyte membrane, after digestion of the C3b by the C3b inactivator. Most lymphoid cells having complement receptors possess both the b and d receptors, however, certain lymphocyte subpopulations, or cells in different differentiation stages show considerable variation in the expression of these receptors (Table 1).

Complement-receptor-bearing lymphocytes are determined by rosetting techniques employing erythrocytes coated with heterologous IgM anti-erythrocyte antibody and complement (Bianco *et al.*, 1970; Bianco, 1976; Ehlenberger and Nussenzweig, 1976; Ross and Polley, 1975, 1976; Winchester and Ross, 1976). These rosettes are called EAC rosettes from the initials of their components (erythrocyte–antibody–complement). Erythrocytes from various sources have been used for EAC-rosette formation. Human erythrocytes are not recommended for EAC complexes because they possess immune adherence receptors (Aiuti *et al.*, 1974) and when coated with complement may rosette among themselves. Usually, sheep erythrocytes are employed and the assay is performed at 37°C (with rotation) to avoid E-rosette formation. They are coated with maximum subagglutinating concentration of rabbit IgM anti-sheep-erythrocyte antibody and either (C5-deficient) mouse serum as a source of complement, or purified human or guinea pig complement (Bianco, 1976; Ehlenberger and Nussenzweig, 1976; Ross and Polley, 1976) as shown in Fig. 5. EAC complexes obtained by addition of mouse serum to EIgM are not specific for either of the C receptors containing variable amounts of EIgMC$\overline{1,4b}$, EIgMC$\overline{1}$, $\overline{4b}$,2a,3b and EIgMC$\overline{1}$, $\overline{4b}$,2a,3d complexes, because of the presence of C4b-C3b inactivator(s) in serum. Using purified complement components, the following EAC complexes can be prepared: (a) EIgMC$\overline{1,4b}$, specific for the CR I or immune adherence or b receptor; (b) EIgMC$\overline{1}$, $\overline{4b}$,2a,3b, that binds to both the CR I (or b) and the CR II (or d) receptors; however, it does not bind to cells bearing only weak C3d receptors and, therefore, cannot be used for the detection of all complement-receptor-bearing lymphocytes; and (c) EIgMC$\overline{1}$, $\overline{4b}$,2a,3d, specific for the CR II or d receptor.

EAC-rosette-forming cells are separated on a preparative scale by centrifugation on Ficoll–Hypaque density cushion in a manner similar to the other rosette-forming cells. Mouse and rat complement-receptor-bearing cells have also been separated by this process (Parish and Hayward, 1974b; Parish, 1975). Information on the stability of EAC complexes—involving weak complement receptors—during the isolation procedure has not been reported.

It should be mentioned that a number of other methods have also been used for the detection of complement receptor bearing lymphocytes. These include immunofluorescence with complement components (Ross and Polley, 1975; Theofilopoulos *et al.*, 1974; Yefenof *et al.*, 1978), use of radio-labeled complement components (Miller *et al.*, 1973), and zymosan particles (Mendes *et al.*, 1974). The latter when mixed with serum activate the

(a) Sheep Erythrocytes (E) + IgM → EIgM $\xrightarrow{C1}$ EIgMC$\overline{1}$ $\xrightarrow{C4}$ EIgMC$\overline{1,4b}$
(binds to the CR I or b receptor)

(b) EIgMC$\overline{1,4b}$ $\xrightarrow{C2}$ EIgMC$\overline{1}$, $\overline{4b}$,2a

$\qquad\qquad$ C3 $\downarrow$

C3a + EIgMC$\overline{1}$, $\overline{4b}$,2a,3b
(binds to both CR I and CR II or b and d receptors)

(c) EIgMC$\overline{1,4b}$ + C4b-C3b inactivator(s) → C3c + EIgMC$\overline{1}$, $\overline{4b}$,2a,3d (binds to CR II or d receptor)

FIGURE 5. Reactions taking place during formation of the various EAC complexes.

C3 through the alternate complement pathway and form ZC complexes which can be used as conventional EAC reagents having longer storage life than erythrocytes.

E. Separation of Human B Lymphocyte Subpopulations by Rosetting Methods

Mouse erythrocytes form spontaneous rosettes with human B lymphocytes bearing IgM or IgD (Stathopoulos and Elliott, 1974; Gupta and Grieco, 1975). These rosettes (5–10% in normal peripheral blood) are presumably a very early B-cell differentiation marker in ontogeny and are independent of surface immunoglobulin, Fc, and complement receptors (Gupta et al., 1976a). Treatment of lymphocytes with neuraminidase permits rosette formation with mouse erythrocytes of all the non-T cells in the peripheral blood [B cells and "third population" (Gupta et al., 1976a)]. Treatment of mouse erythrocytes with papain permits the formation of rosettes stable enough to be used in the separation procedures on Ficoll–Triosil. The rosetting fraction contains all or most of the B cells whereas the nonrosetting population contains 90% E-rosette-forming cells (Zola, 1977).

Human B lymphocytes can be detected or isolated by a direct immunocytoadhesion technique, using SRBC coated, via $CrCl_3$, with goat anti-human $F(ab')_2$ (Giuliano et al., 1974) or with rabbit anti-human light-chain antibodies (Strelkauskas et al., 1975). This conjugation procedure, via $CrCl_3$, will be discussed in the next paragraph. Anti-immunoglobulin antibody-coated SRBC form rosettes with B lymphocytes, which are subsequently separated by centrifugation on Ficoll–Hypaque density cushion. B lymphocytes are recovered from the pellet after lysis of the erythrocytes by Tris-ammonium chloride (Strelkauskas et al., 1975).

F. Separation of Rodent T and B Lymphocytes by Rosetting Methods

Rosetting techniques have also been applied for the separation of T and B mouse and rat lymphocytes (Parish et al., 1974; Parish and Hayward, 1974a,b,c; Parish, 1975). For this type of separation, rabbit anti-mouse- or anti-rat-Ig antibody is reacted with mouse or rat lymphocytes, respectively, and the latter are rosetted with SRBC coated (via $CrCl_3$) with sheep or horse anti-rabbit-Ig antibody (IgG fraction). The rosetting cells are subsequently separated by centrifugation on Ficoll–Hypaque [density 1.09 g/cm^3 (Parish et al., 1974)] and contain all the precursors of antibody forming cells (B lymphocytes), few helper cells, and theta antigen-bearing lymphocytes, but no MLC-responding cells. The nonrosetting cells—

recovered from the interface—contain almost all the theta-positive cells including the bulk of the helper cells and the proliferating and cytotoxic cells in MLC. The exact mechanism of the binding of immunoglobulin to sheep erythrocytes via $CrCl_3$ is poorly understood. Detailed methodological aspects of this reaction have been reported by several investigators (Gold and Fudenberg, 1967; Parish and Hayward, 1974a; Kofler and Wick, 1977; Ling et al., 1977). Similar methodology has been applied for the coating of SRBC with goat anti-human $F(ab')_2$, which is useful in the detection and isolation of human B lymphocytes (Giuliano et al., 1974; Strelkauskas et al., 1975).

Sheep erythrocytes coated with rat anti-SRBC antibody were employed for the separation of Fc-receptor-positive lymphocytes on Ficoll–Hypaque (Parish and Hayward, 1974a,b). Furthermore, an additional rosetting procedure has been reported for the enumeration of I-J-positive lymphocytes (suppressor cells) in the mouse (Parish and McKenzie, 1977) and of murine lymphocytes that react with various alloantisera (Parish and McKenzie, 1978). Immunoglobulin-negative mouse lymphocytes were incubated with mouse anti-I-J serum followed by the addition of SRBC coated with sheep anti-mouse-Ig antibody. The formed rosettes permit the direct visualization of the I-J-positive cells (Parish and McKenzie, 1977). The small numbers of I-J-positive cells (less than 5%) discouraged attempts to isolate these cells on a preparative scale.

Protein-A-coated erythrocytes (via $CrCl_3$) have also been applied to the detection, enumeration, and preparative separation of lymphocytes reacted with allo- or xenoantisera (Ghetie et al., 1974, 1975; Dorval et al., 1974; Sandrin et al., 1978; Johnson, 1977). Following rosette formation, rosette-forming cells and nonrosetting lymphocytes are separated by centrifugation on Ficoll–Hypaque density cushion (Ghetie et al., 1975). Using this methodology (Fig. 6) Sandrin et al. (1978) were able to detect alloantibodies to H-2 (including Ia specificities), Ly-1, 2, 4, 5, 6, 7, and Thy-1 antigens bound to the surface of the lymphocytes. This procedure is reported to be superior to certain complement-mediated cytotoxic assays (Sandrin et al., 1978).

Furthermore, rosetting with sheep erythrocytes has been employed for the separation of specific antigen (e.g., SRBC)-binding mouse lymphocytes (Osoba, 1970; Brody, 1970; Wilson, 1973) with the disadvantage that the isolated cells are specific not for a single antigenic determinant but for several.

G. Other Spontaneous Erythrocyte Rosettes

Erythrocytes from a number of species form spontaneous rosettes with human and/or animal lymphocyte subpopulations. These rosettes may be

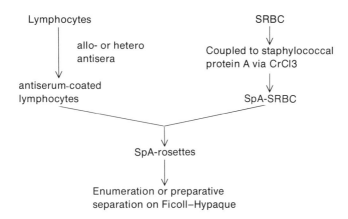

FIGURE 6. Rosetting using antisera against a surface marker and protein-A-coated SRBC.

proven useful for the separation of such lymphocyte subpopulations. Rhesus monkey erythrocytes form spontaneous rosettes with human T lymphocytes (Lohrmann and Novikous, 1974). In contrast, Japanese monkey (*Macaca speciosa*) erythrocytes, form spontaneous rosettes with B lymphocytes and "third population" cells (Pellegrino *et al.*, 1975b). However, these observations have been recently challenged by other investigators who found that monkey red blood cell rosettes are not a specific marker for human T or B cells (Patel *et al.*, 1978).

Human thymocytes and T lymphocytes from peripheral blood (3%–8%) and other lymphoid organs form spontaneous rosettes with autologous erythrocytes, the so-called autorosettes. These autorosette-forming cells may include a subpopulation of less mature cells (Baxley *et al.*, 1973; Sandilands *et al.*, 1974; Charreire and Bach, 1974; Kaplan, 1975; Gluckman and Montambault, 1975; Yu, 1975). Treatment of peripheral blood lymphocytes with Con A resulted in significant increase of autorosette-forming cells (with 2 μg/ml of Con A, 36% RFC; with 10 μg/ml of Con A, 56% RFC). These cells were separated on a preparative scale by centrifugation on a Ficoll–Hypaque density cushion (Fournier and Charreire, 1978). Whether or not these autorosette-forming cells represent a functionally distinct lymphocyte subpopulation remains to be established.

Rabbit red blood cells form spontaneous rosettes with a large proportion (45%) of human thymocytes and very few (1%) with peripheral blood lymphocytes (Yu and Gale, 1977). Finally, T cells from a number of animal species form rosettes with heterologous erythrocytes (Wahl *et al.*, 1976). Although additional studies are required for the immunological characterization of these rosetting cells in animals, their usefulness in separating functionally distinct lymphocyte subpopulations is apparent.

III. AFFINITY CHROMATOGRAPHY OF CELLS AND CELLULAR IMMUNOABSORBENT METHODS

A. Introduction

Affinity chromatography and cellular immunoabsorbent methods (including cell monolayers) offer another approach for the isolation, depletion, or enrichment of lymphocyte subpopulations. They were first introduced for depletion of specific antigen-binding cells (Wigzell and Andersson, 1969), and they are currently used for the separation or depletion of a variety of lymphocyte subpopulations including B lymphocytes (Wigzell *et al.*, 1972; Schlossman and Hudson, 1973; Chess *et al.*, 1974a; Mage *et al.*, 1977), complement receptor bearing cells (Jondal *et al.*, 1973), Fc-receptor-bearing cells (Jondal *et al.*, 1973; Kedar *et al.*, 1974), specific antigen- or hapten-binding lymphocytes (Wigzell *et al.*, 1972; Haas and Layton, 1975; Haas, 1975; Nossal and Pike, 1976), and cytotoxic T lymphocytes (Berke and Levey, 1972; Brondz and Snegiröva, 1971; Neefe and Sachs, 1976).

The affinity methods employ solid-phase supportive materials to which are chemically bound (by covalent linkage) or absorbed (by adherence) molecules (usually specific antibodies) that bind to cell surface antigens, receptors or markers selectively expressed on functionally distinct lymphocyte subpopulations. A number of materials have been used as solid-phase immunoabsorbents including glass beads, polymethacrylic plastic beads (Degalan), (Wigzell and Andersson, 1969; Wigzell, 1976a,b), cross-linked dextrans, e.g., Sephadex G-200 (Schlossman and Hudson, 1973; Chess *et al.*, 1974a; Chess and Schlossman, 1976), acrylamide (Truffa-Bachi and Wofsy, 1970), polystyrene plastic dishes (Kedar *et al.*, 1974; Mage *et al.*, 1977), and Sepharose (Scott, 1976b; Casali and Perussia, 1977; Ghetie *et al.*, 1978). These materials, after proper treatment, exhibit minimum or significantly reduced nonspecific retention in comparison to the selective binding of the cell types of interest. They are used either in the form of affinity chromatography columns where the nonadherent cells are moving downward by gravity, or as flat surface immunoabsorbents (e.g., petri dishes) where the nonadherent cells are carefully removed by decantation and washing.

B. Separation of Immunoglobulin-Positive and Immunoglubulin-Negative Lymphocytes by Affinity Chromatography Methods

Rodent or human immunoglobulin-bearing cells have been depleted from lymphoid populations and subsequently isolated (in certain cases) by anti-immunoglubulin/immunoglubulin-coated glass or plastic (Degalan) bead columns (Wigzell *et al.*, 1972; Binz *et al.*, 1974; Wigzell *et al.*, 1972; Wigzell, 1976a; Kondorosi *et al.* 1977). The glass or plastic beads are coated (by adsorption) with the immunoglobulin of the cell species to be separated followed by a second coating with heterologous anti-Ig antibody at high concentrations. For example, columns prepared for isolation of rat lymphocytes are initially coated with rat immunoglobulin, followed by a second coating with rabbit anti-rat Ig. The use of high concentrations of the heterologous anti-Ig antibody is necessary, so that the latter binds to the Ig-coated beads only through one of the antigen-binding sites. The other site is free to combine with the Ig-positive cells. Such a binding mediated through specific but weak interacting forces delays the flow of these cells through the column, so that they can be retained by the beads by stronger, but nonspecific, adsorption forces as discussed by Wigzell and Andersson (1971) and Wigzell (1976a). The fact that mechanical elution is sufficient for the recovery of the bound cells support the suggested mechanism of retention (Wigzell and Andersson, 1971).

Alternatively, lymphocytes coated with high concentrations of anti-immunoglobulin antibody are passed through Ig-coated columns. Ig-positive cells are retained by binding to the Ig-coated beads through one of the antigen-binding sites of anti-Ig. This antigen-binding site remains free because an excess of anti-Ig antibody is used for coating of the cells. The double-coating techniques are reported to be superior to the use of anti-Ig coated columns (Wigzell, 1976a,b). However, these anti-immunoglobulin/immunoglobulin-coated glass or plastic bead methods have several advantages and disadvantages. Among the former are complete, or almost complete, removal of Ig-bearing cells and ability to handle a large number of cells. Among the latter, the nonspecific retention of cells appears to be of importance. It results in poor enrichment of Ig-bearing lymphocytes in the eluted cell fractions, unless, the more "sticky" cells are removed in advance by passage through normal serum coated columns. By this means highly purified B cells can be prepared (Wigzell *et al.*, 1972). Another disadvantage of the method is binding of the cells through their Fc receptors when intact antibody molecules are used (Perlmann *et al.*, 1973).

Sephadex G-200 (cross-linked dextran) is another material extensively used for separation of B and non-B lymphocytes. Schlossman and Hudson (1973) employed a Sephadex G-200 conjugated rabbit anti-mouse-Fab column for the separation of mouse spleen Ig-positive and Ig-negative cells. T and null lymphocytes pass through the column whereas B lymphocytes are retained. The latter are recovered by digestion of the Sephadex G-200 immunoabsorbent by dextranase. Similarly, Sephadex G-200 rabbit anti-human-F(ab)$_2$ columns have been employed for the preparative separation of human B and non-B lymphocytes (Chess *et al.*, 1974a,b,c; Chess and

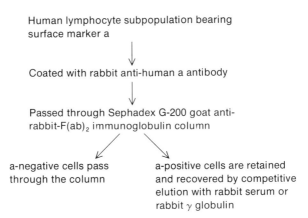

FIGURE 7.   Separation of cells bearing specific surface markers or differentiation antigens by affinity chromatography.

Schlossman, 1976b, 1977). B lymphocytes bind to these immunoabsorbents; both T and null cells pass through. The latter can be further fractionated to T and null cells by E-rosetting. The bound B lymphocytes can be recovered from the column by competitive elution with human immunoglobulin, and contain less than 2% E-rosette-positive cells and higher than 98% immunoglobulin-positive lymphocytes. Sephadex G-200 itself is reported as a "near-perfect filter for human lymphocytes and monocytes" (Chess and Schlossman, 1977) with negligible, if any, nonspecific retention of the cells (Schlossman and Hudson, 1973), permitting high yield and purity of recovered bound B lymphocytes. In addition, the majority of the Fc receptor-bearing cells do not bind to these columns. However, the possible binding to Sephadex G-200 anti-F(ab)$_2$ columns of the so-called L cells, non-B lymphocytes which bear cytophilic IgG in their surface (Lobo *et al.*, 1975; Winchester *et al.*, 1975; Horowitz and Lobo, 1975; Ault *et al.*, 1976), has not been given particular attention.

This methodology can be used for the isolation of any type of lymphoid cells bearing surface antigens which can be recognized by specific antisera (Fig. 7). Thus, p23,30-positive (a human Ia-like antigen) cells were isolated from a null cell population. Immunoglobulin-negative cells were coated with rabbit anti-p23,30 and subsequently passed through a Sephadex G-200 goat anti-rabbit Ig column. The retained cells—recovered by competitive elusion with rabbit γ-globulin—were shown to be p23,30-positive (Chess *et al.*, 1976a). The same methodology has been applied by Cantor *et al.* (1976) for positive selection of Ly-2$^+$ cells. Spleen or lymph node mouse T lymphocytes, prepared by nylon wool columns, were coated with anti-Ly-2 serum and subsequently passed through a Sephadex G-200 rabbit anti-mouse-Fab column. Only the Ly-2$^+$ cells were retained by the column and recovered by competitive elution with normal mouse serum.

In another method (Mage et al., 1977), polystyrene tissue culture dishes coated with purified goat anti-mouse immunoglobulin were employed for the separation of Ig-positive and Ig-negative cells. Goat anti-mouse antibody from a hyperimmune serum was purified by affinity chromatography and adsorbed to polystyrene tissue culture dishes by overnight incubation. Spleen lymphocytes were fractionated by these immunoabsorbents by incubation at room temperature for 1 h. The nonadherent cell populations were at least 95% Ig-negative, responded in mixed lymphocyte culture, and possessed the effector cells in graft-vs-host (GvH) and cell-mediated cytotoxicity (CTL). Ig-positive lymphocytes were recovered from the plates by mechanical agitation and competitive elution with anti-Ig antibody. In this case the recovered cells were at least 94% Ig-positive and exhibited a viability of 90% or higher. This technique can handle high quantities of cells, up to 2×10^8 per single 10-mm diameter polystyrene petri plate.

Staphylococcal protein A (SpA) covalently linked to Sepharose 6MB (SpA–Sepharose 6MB) is another immunoabsorbent used for the separation of immunoglobulin-positive and immunoglobulin-negative cells from mouse spleen (Ghetie et al., 1978). This method is based on the reaction of protein A with the Fc region of most mammalian IgG immunoglobulins. The interaction between SpA and rabbit IgG is quite strong (affinity constant 10^8–10^9) so that lymphocytes coated with rabbit IgG are retained by the SpA-coated columns. Sepharose 6MB itself exhibits negligible nonspecific retention of lymphocytes. Mouse spleen lymphocytes coated with rabbit anti-mouse-Ig antibody (IgG fraction) have been fractionated by passage through SpA–Sepharose 6MB columns. The nonretained cells were shown to be T lymphocytes (up to 70%) and null cells. The retained cells recovered either by mechanical agitation or competitive elution with dog IgG, were Ig-positive. However, complete removal of the Ig-positive cells requires repetitive passage of the nonretained cells through the column. An advantage of this method is that it can be used for the separation of practically any lymphocyte subpopulation coated with IgG antibody specific to one of its surface markers.

Affinity chromatograph on antifluorescein antibody-Sepharose 4B columns (Scott, 1976a,b) is another technique for the separation of human B lymphocytes (Johnson et al., 1977). Purified antifluorescein KLH was conjugated to Sepharose 4B by standard procedures (Scott, 1976b). Human peripheral blood lymphocytes were coated with fluorescein-conjugated goat anti-human immunoglobulin and passed through the column. Fourteen per cent of the cells which passed through the column and 75% of the retained cells (recovered by competitive elution with fluoresceinated BSA) were immunoglobulin-positive (Johnson *et al.*, 1977). The antifluorescein-antibody-coated columns were initially developed for the isolation of antigen-specific B lymphocytes (Scott, 1976a).

C3-reacted Sepharose columns have been used for the separation of complement-receptor-bearing human lymphocytes (Casali and Perussia, 1977). The retained complement-receptor-positive lymphocytes were eluted from the column with a rabbit antiserum to human C3. B lymphocytes isolated by this procedure will be contaminated by a small number of third-population cells bearing complement receptors. Complement-receptor-bearing lymphocytes have been fractionated also by Degalan columns coated with aggregated immunoglobulin and complement components (Wigzell *et al.*, 1972a).

C. Separation of Fc-Receptor-Bearing Lymphocytes by Affinity Methods

Fc-receptor-bearing lymphocytes have been depleted from lymphocyte populations by adsorption with Degalan beads coated with antigen–antibody complexes (Basten *et al.*, 1972). However, the efficiency of such a depletion has been challenged (Karpf *et al.*, 1975).

Kedar *et al.* (1974) contributed another interesting method for the isolation of Fc-receptor-positive cells. Polystyrene petri dishes, treated with poly-L-lysine, were coated with sheep erythrocytes and subsequently with anti-sheep-erythrocyte antibody (Kennedy and Axelrad, 1971), as shown in Fig. 8. Fc-receptor-bearing cells adhere to these erythrocyte-antibody monolayers and can be recovered by lysis of the sheep erythrocytes with Tris-ammonium chloride. The binding of human Fc-receptor-positive cells to immobilized antigen–antibody complexes is followed by significant changes in cell shape and morphology within a few minutes after binding (Alexander and Henkart, 1976). These changes are presumably due to the modulation of the Fc receptor of the cells as discussed previously for the rosetting techniques. A comparable method for the separation of Fc-receptor-bearing cells has been described by Targan and Jondal (1978). The latter employed human IgG-rabbit anti-human-IgG-coated plastic tissue culture dishes (monolayer immune complexes) for the fractionation of human peripheral blood lymphocytes that are effectors in ADCC and NK cytotoxic assays.

The presence of Fc receptors in a number of lymphoid cell types decreases the capacity of these methods to separate functionally distinct lymphocyte subpopulations when unfractionated lymphocytes are separated. However, these techniques are useful for the separation of Fc-recep-

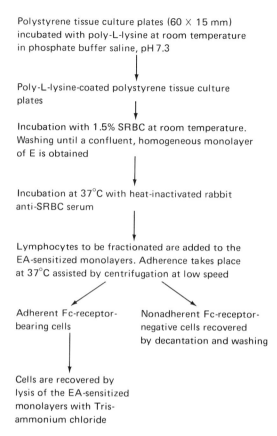

Polystyrene tissue culture plates (60 × 15 mm) incubated with poly-L-lysine at room temperature in phosphate buffer saline, pH 7.3

↓

Poly-L-lysine-coated polystyrene tissue culture plates

↓

Incubation with 1.5% SRBC at room temperature. Washing until a confluent, homogeneous monolayer of E is obtained

↓

Incubation at 37°C with heat-inactivated rabbit anti-SRBC serum

↓

Lymphocytes to be fractionated are added to the EA-sensitized monolayers. Adherence takes place at 37°C assisted by centrifugation at low speed

Adherent Fc-receptor-bearing cells

Nonadherent Fc-receptor-negative cells recovered by decantation and washing

↓

Cells are recovered by lysis of the EA-sensitized monolayers with Tris-ammonium chloride

FIGURE 8. Separation of Fc-receptor-bearing cells by EA-sensitized monolayers, as described by Kedar *et al.* (1974).

tor-bearing cells from prepurified lymphocyte populations by other methods (e.g., T cells).

D. Separation of Specific Antigen-Binding Lymphocytes by Affinity Methods

Cellular immunoabsorbent methods for the isolation of specific antigen binding cells were first introduced by Wigzell and Andersson (1969). Plastic or glass bead columns coated with antigen were used for the depletion of antigen-specific plaque-forming cells and immunological memory cells from mouse lymphoid cell populations. The observation that free antigen blocks the retention of these cells supported Burnet's clonal selection theory (Burnet, 1959). Similar observations were made with specific hapten-binding cells (Wigzell and Mäkelä, 1970). Although such columns were efficient for the depletion of specific antigen-binding lymphocytes, the recovery of these cells in a highly purified state was problematic because of the presence of considerable numbers of contaminating other cells, retained by nonspecific absorption by the glass or plastic beads (Wigzell and Mäkelä, 1970; Wigzell, 1971). These problems were significantly reduced by the introduction of other materials as solid-phase immunoabsorbents. Truffa-Bachi and Wofsy (1970) introduced polyacrylamide beads as an efficient solid-phase matrix for the depletion and recovery of specific antigen-binding cells (β-lactoside hapten groups). Hapten-specific-binding cells, eluted by free hapten, were significantly enriched in indirect plaque-forming cells against the hapten (Wofsy et al., 1971). Recovery of specific hapten-binding cells, by free hapten, was also reported by Choi et al. (1974). These authors used polystyrene tubes coated with rabbit anti-p-azobenzoate antibody and KLH-p-azobenzoate. However, other reports (Wigzell, 1970; Edelman et al., 1971) have indicated that cells once bound to immunoabsorbents could not be recovered by free-antigen elution. Edelman and his collaborators (Edelman et al., 1971) employed antigens covalently linked to nylon strings of fibers. Specific antigen-binding cells were recovered by plucking the fibers.

Haas and co-workers reported a method for the separation and recovery of specific antigen binding cells using hapten-conjugated gelatin in plastic petri dishes (Haas et al., 1974; Haas and Layton, 1975; Haas, 1975). The attractive feature of this technique is that the hapten–gelatin conjugates form insoluble matrixes at low temperatures (4°C) to which specific antigen-binding cells are bound. The latter are recovered by incubation of the dishes at 37°C where the hapten–gelatin matrix melts. The remaining gelatin is removed from the surface of the specific antigen-binding cells by collagenase treatment. Using these procedures, Haas and Layton (1975) and Haas (1975) were able to enrich 300-fold anti-NIP antibody-forming cell progenitors and 100-fold anti-DNP antibody-forming cell progenitors. Nossal and Pike (1976) applied this method in combination with micromanipulation techniques of single lymphocytes and microcultures of small numbers of cells for studies on anti-hapten antibody-forming clones.

The same investigators (Nossal and Pike, 1978) reported an improved procedure for the fractionation and stimulation in vitro of hapten-specific B lymphocytes. This method (Fig. 9) consisted of two successive hapten–gelatin fractionation cycles followed by an additional fractionation step by rosetting using hapten-coated SRBC. These three successive cycles of fractionation (two of NIP-gelatin and one of NIP–rosetting) separated a population of cells with average frequency of anti-NIP precursors of 0.28, whereas a single NIP-gelatin fractionation cycle provided a 0.04 frequency.

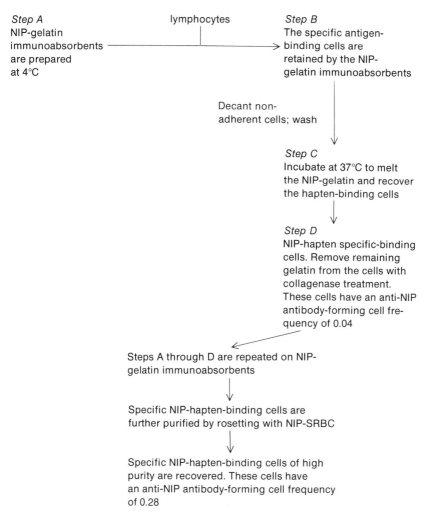

FIGURE 9.   Separation of specific hapten-binding cells according to Nossal and Pike (1978).

In another report Nossal *et al.* (1978) used one cycle fluorescein-gelatin fractionation followed by electronic cell sorting for the enrichment of hapten-specific B lymphocytes. After cell sorting, the cells bearing strong fluorescence ($\approx 10\%$) exhibited a 1 : 8 frequency of plaque-forming clones which was five times higher than cells enriched only by hapten–gelatin fractionation. Less fluorescent cohorts of cells showed gradually lower plaque-forming cell precursor frequency and produced antibody with lower avidity for the antigen; a finding which is in agreement with the clonal selection theory.

Another method for the separation of specific antigen-binding cells has been described by Scott (1976b). It employs fluoresceinated antigens and antifluorescein Ig-Sephadex G-200 or Sepharose 4B columns. The cells to be separated are incubated *in vivo* or *in vitro* with FITC-conjugated specific antigen and subsequently pass through an anti-FITC antibody column. Specific antigen binding cells are retained by the column and eluted with a fluoresceinated unrelated protein. The isolated specific antigen-binding cells have been shown to be fully immunocompetent. The procedure has also been applied to the isolation of polymerized flagellin-binding B cells as well as TNP-specific B lymphocytes (Scott, 1976a, b).

Highly enriched specific antigen-binding cells have also been obtained by using the fluorescence-activated cell sorter (Julius *et al.*, 1972; Julius and Herzenberg, 1974; Scott, 1976a). The method is limited to a few users only, by the high cost of the apparatus. The number of cells that can separate within reasonable amount of time is relatively small and, of course, fluorescent-labeled haptens or antigens are required.

A procedure to isolate enriched populations of antigen-specific suppressor cells has been described by Okumura *et al.* (1977). They employed KLH-coated Sephadex G-200 columns. Specific KLH-suppressor T cells from KLH-immunized mice were specifically bound to the columns at 37°C and subsequently eluted with cold medium. A 100-fold enrichment in specific suppressor activity was achieved by this method. The isolated antigen-specific suppressor T cells were I-J+, Ly-2+,3+ and FcR⁻ T lymphocytes (Okumura *et al.*, 1977). Helper T lymphocytes did not bind to these columns. An additional method for enriching specific suppressor T lymphocytes was reported by Taniguchi and Miller (1977) employing antigen (HGG)-coated tissue culture grade polystyrene petri dishes prepared in a way similar to the one described by Mage *et al.* (1977) for the isolation of B lymphocytes.

E. Separation of Cytotoxic T Lymphocytes by Cellular Immunoabsorbent Methods

Absorption on target cell monolayers has been extensively used for the separation of specific cytotoxic lymphocytes (CTL). These methods are based on the presence of specific antigen receptors for target cells on the surface of CTLs. The binding of sensitized xenoreactive T lymphocytes to target cells was first reported by Wilson (1965). Further evidence was obtained by microcinematography methods (Ginsburg *et al.*, 1969). Based on the above findings, Brondz and Snegiröva (1971) employed macrophage monolayers grown on flat-faced tubes to retain specific cytotoxic T lymphocytes from *in vivo* sensitized mice (Brondz, 1972). Subsequently, other investigators used allogeneic fibroblast monolayers in petri dishes to remove specific cytotoxic T cells (Berke and Levey, 1972; Altman *et al.*, 1973; Bach *et al.*, 1973; Mage and McHugh, 1973). Absorption of previously sensitized lymphocyte populations with monolayers selectively eliminated or significantly decreased the specific cytolytic activity. The nonadherent cells were readily sensitized to allogeneic cells, histoin-compatible to the monolayer target cells, but not to cells syngeneic to the monolayer. Specific cytotoxic T lymphocytes retained by the cell monolayers could be recovered by trypsinization and subsequent separation on albumin gradients (Golstein *et al.*, 1971; Berke and Levey, 1972), or by addition of EDTA (Berke and Levey, 1972; Chisholm and Ford, 1978).

Another cellular immunoabsorbent technique has been introduced by Stulting and Berke (1973). They employed tumor cell monolayers attached to plastic petri dishes by polylysine. This method is a modification of the one reported by Kennedy and Axelrad (1971) for the preparation of red blood cell monolayers using poly-L-lysine-coated plastic tissue-culture plates. The introduction of the poly-L-lysine coating method eliminated the need to use exclusively cells forming adherent monolayers in culture. Tumor cells, spleen lymphocytes, as well as other lymphoid or nonlymphoid cells can be used for the formation of cellular immunoabsorbents. Using this methodology cytotoxic lymphocytes can be depleted from a population of sensitized cells as described in several reports (Stulting and Berke, 1973; Mage and McHugh, 1975; Lonai *et al.*, 1973; Neefe and Sachs, 1976). The cytotoxic cells recovered (by EDTA treatment) are usually contaminated by 15–25% of detached monolayer cells (Stulting and Berke, 1973; Neefe and Sachs, 1976). Although cytotoxic effector cells are retained by these immunoabsorbents, GvH-reactive lymphocytes cannot be depleted (Mage and McHugh, 1973; Clark and Kimura, 1973; Stulting and Berke, 1974; Rubin, 1975; Neefe and Sachs, 1976; Chisholm and Ford, 1978) with the exception of some reports (Lonai *et al.*, 1973; Mage and McHugh, 1975) where partial depletion under certain circumstances was achieved. The failure of the majority of immunoabsorbents to retain the GvH-reactive cells may be explained, at least in the mouse system, by the fact that they may recognize lymphocyte-defined (Ia) determinants whereas the cytotoxic cells recognize serologically-defined determinants (Cantor and Boyse, 1977; Alter *et al.*, 1971).

Recently Singer *et al.* (1978) reported another method for the selective depletion and enrichment of specific cytotoxic T lymphocytes using anti-fluorescein affinity columns. Peritoneal exudate cells from BALB/c mice, immunized with EL-4 ascites lymphoma, were mixed with EL-4 cells labeled directly with fluorescein and passed through an anti-fluorescein column (horse anti-FITC-KLH). The fluoresceinated EL-4 tumor cells having cytotoxic lymphocytes bound to them, were retained by the column and subsequently eluted with EDTA. However, although the nonadherent cells were almost completely depleted from CTL activity, the recovered cells were not always enriched in specific CTLs. An advantage of this method is the low contamination of the eluted cytotoxic lymphocytes by absorbing cells (less than 5%) (Singer *et al.*, 1978).

IV. ELIMINATION OF LYMPHOCYTE SUBPOPULATIONS BY ANTISERA PLUS COMPLEMENT TREATMENT

In vitro treatment of lymphoid cell populations with antiserum specific for one of their surface markers and complement is a popular and convenient method for the negative selection and elimination of functionally distinct lymphocyte subpopulations. Two protocols are currently used. The one-step protocol where the lymphocytes are incubated with antiserum in the presence of complement, and the two- step protocol where the lymphocytes are incubated with antisera (usually for 30–60 min), washed, and then incubated with complement (at 37°C for 30 min). The two-step protocol is suggested when antisera with suspected soluble antigen–antibody complexes that fix the complement are used. Antisera used in the complement-mediated cytolysis methods should be specific and have high titre. Rabbit or guinea pig serum is usually employed as a nontoxic complement source. Toxicity of the complement can be eliminated by absorption with agar (Cohen and Schlesinger, 1970).

This method is extensively employed for tissue typing and detection of alloantigens (Boyse *et al.*, 1964) and for the isolation of functionally distinct lymphocyte subpopulations on a preparative scale. Dead cells (visualized by a dye exclusion viability assay) can be removed by centrifugation on Ficoll–Hypaque density cushion (Bøyum, 1968; Davidson and Parish, 1975), centrifugation on a dense albumin layer at neutral pH (Shortman *et al.*, 1972), or by using the low ionic strength filtration method of von Boehmer and Shortman (1973). A large number of applications of this methodology are reported in the literature. Representative are the elimination of T lymphocytes by anti-theta serum (Raff, 1970; Takahashi *et al.*, 1971), of B lymphocytes by anti-immunoglobulin serum (Takahashi *et al.*, 1971; Miller *et al.*, 1972; McArthur *et al.*, 1971; Ryser and Vassalli, 1974; Gmelig-Meyling *et al.*, 1974; Potash and Knopf, 1978) and Ly-1+ or Ly-2,3+ cells by treatment with the appropriate anti-Ly antiserum (Cantor and Boyse, 1975). A disadvantage of this method is that the eliminated population of cells is not recovered.

V. ELIMINATION OF SPECIFIC LYMPHOCYTE SUBPOPULATIONS BY SELECTIVE INCORPORATION OF HIGH-SPECIFIC-ACTIVITY RADIOISOTOPES ("SUICIDE" METHODS)

Methods for inactivation of specific antigen-binding lymphocytes by selective incorporation of radioisotope of high specific activity ("suicide" methods) have been used primarily in studies involving specific antigen-binding to lymphoid cells, as well as responding cells in mixed lymphocyte culture. Incubation of lymphocytes *in vitro* with radio-iodinated antigen of very high specific activity eliminates or greatly reduces their capacity to respond to this antigen upon transfer to irradiated syngeneic recipients in both primary and secondary adoptive immune responses. The ability of the injected lymphocytes to transfer immunity for other antigens was not affected (Ada and Byrd, 1969; Golan and Borel, 1972; Roelants and Askonas, 1971). Depletion of the antigen-binding cells has been shown to be antigen or hapten specific. These experiments taken together with results on the binding of radiolabeled antigen to very small proportions of lymphocytes (in the range of 0.02–0.5% of the total) were the first experimental evidence in support of the clonal selection theory (Naor and Sulitzean, 1967; Byrd and Ada, 1969).

Zoschke and Bach (1971a,b) introduced the 5-bromodeoxyuridine (BUdR) method (Djordjevic and Szybalski, 1960; Puck and Kao, 1967) for the inactivation of specific T lymphocytes responding in mixed lymphocyte culture to a certain histocompatibility haplotype. BUdR was added to human mixed lymphocyte cultures immediately after mixing the responding and stimulating cells. Additions of BUdR were repeated every 24 h for the first 96 h in culture to a final concentration of 1×10^{-5} M. The lymphocytes were exposed to visible and near visible light, washed, and used as responding cells. Response of lymphocytes to the stimulating haplotype was completely abolished whereas response to third-party cells was unaffected. The method is based on the incorporation of the thymidine analog BUdR into the DNA of the dividing cells (e.g., the clones responding to the initial allogeneic cell-stimulating haplotype) and inactivation of these cells by exposure to visible or near visible light. Zoschke and Bach (1970) employed this method for the selective elimination of specific antigen-binding cells.

VI. SEPARATION OF LYMPHOCYTE SUBPOPULATIONS BY THE USE OF LECTINS

A number of lectins have been shown to bind reversibly to certain lymphocyte subpopulations. The binding is mediated by surface receptors of glycoprotein or other molecular nature with carbohydrate residues specific for each lectin, as shown by competitive inhibition experiments. On the basis of this selective and reversible binding, methods for the preparative isolation of lymphocyte subpopulations have been developed employing a number of different lectins.

Hammarström *et al.* (1973) reported the binding of *Helix pomatia* A hemagglutinin to human T lymphocytes after treatment of the latter with neuraminidase. The same group of workers fractionated neuraminidase-treated human peripheral blood leukocytes using *Helix pomatia* A hemagglutinin conjugated to Sepharose 6MB. The cells ($\approx 10\%$) which passed through the column (HP-negative cells) were 50% to 55% immunoglobulin and complement-receptor-positive cells contaminated only with few E-rosette-forming cells (approximately 30% of the total). A second cell fraction (about 10%) was recovered from the column by competitive elution with 0.1 mg/ml N-acetyl-D-galactosamine. The composition of this fraction was mixed. The majority of the HP-positive cells ($\approx 45\%$) were recovered by subsequent elution with 1.0 mg/ml of N-acetyl-D-galactosamine. This fraction was highly enriched in E-rosette-forming cells with a 10% contamination of immunoglobulin-bearing lymphocytes (Hellström *et al.*, 1976). Using the same type of *Helix pomatia*-Sepharose column and the same elution procedures, Haller *et al.* (1978) were able to fractionate neuraminidase-treated mouse spleen lymphocytes according to their affinity for the lectin. The majority of the B lymphocytes were HP-negative cells and passed through the column whereas T lymphocytes were HP-positive and eluted with 1.0 mg/ml of N-acetyl-D-galactosamine. It is of interest that natural killer effector cells were shown to be HP-positive. In another report Axelsson *et al.* (1978) reported the isolation of a HP-binding surface glycoprotein with molecular weight of 130,000 from thymus-derived mouse lymphocytes. This molecule was not found on normal adult mouse B cells. Human T lymphocytes and T leukemia cell lines possess a HP-binding protein of molecular weight 150,000 absent from B lymphocytes at certain differentiation stages (Axelsson *et al.*, 1978).

Wheat-germ agglutinin has also been employed for the fractionation of human T lymphocytes (Hellström *et al.*, 1976). This nonmitogenic lectin is specific for a sequence of three β-(1→4)-linked N-acetyl-D-glucosamine (D-GNAC) residues (Nagata and Burger, 1974; Goldstein *et al.*, 1975) and binds to all lymphocytes, but with different affinity (Karsenti *et al.*, 1975; Boldt *et al.*, 1975; Hellström *et al.*, 1976). Using a wheat-germ agglutinin-conjugated Sephadex G-200 column, Hellström *et al.* (1976) were able to separate two human T lymphocyte populations starting from purified T lymphocytes. High-affinity WGA-binding cells represented 20% of the T cells and were recovered by competitive elution with D-GNAC. Low-affinity WGA-binding cells were passed through the column, or were eluted with buffer. The two populations differed in their responses toward the mitogenic lectins leukoagglutinin (La) (from *Phaseolus vulgaris*) and Con A.

Reisner *et al.* (1976a) used peanut agglutinin (PNA, highly specific for residues of D-galactose) for the separation of mouse thymocytes into two subpopulations (i.e., PNA-positive and PNA-negative cells) by agglutination with the lectin and dissociation of the agglutinated lymphocytes with D-galactose (Lotan *et al.*, 1975). Thymocytes were incubated at room temperature for short periods of time with PNA and the mixture was layered on top of a heat-inactivated fetal calf serum. Within 30 min the PNA-positive cells sedimented to the bottom of the layer whereas unagglutinated cells remained at the interface. Single cell suspensions were recovered from the agglutinated cells by dissociation with D-galactose. The agglutinated cell population (PNA-positive cells) represented approximately 90% of the total thymocytes, responded to Con A but not to PHA, failed to induce GvH reaction and contained cells with high levels of thy-antigen and low H-2. In contrast, the unagglutinated cell population (5–10% of the total thymocytes) responded to both Con A and PHA, induced a vigorous GvH reaction, and contained cells with low thy-antigen content and high H-2. In addition to thymocyte binding, peanut agglutinin binds to small proportions of other lymphoid cells such as spleen (5%), lymph node (15%), and bone marrow cells ($\approx 16\%$) (London *et al.*, 1978). Reisner *et al.* (1976b) were able to separate mouse spleen T and B lymphocytes on the basis of their differential agglutinability to soybean lectin followed by dissociation of the agglutinated cell population by D-galactose. The agglutinated cell fraction contained 5–8% theta-positive cells and 83% immunoglobulin-positive lymphocytes. The nonagglutinated cell fraction contained 78% thy-positive cells with only 5% immunoglobulin-bearing cells (Reisner *et al.*, 1976b).

In another communication, Reisner *et al.* (1978) reported that fractionation of murine bone marrow or spleen cells by peanut and soybean agglutinin yielded a cell population depleted of GvH effector cells and enriched in hemopoietic stem cells. This cell population reconstituted successfully lethally irradiated allogeneic mice, without causing GvH disease.

VII. CONCLUSIONS

In cell separation the method of choice has to fulfill certain criteria. The most important is the ability to separate functionally distinct lymphocyte subpopulations with minimum contamination from other cell types, while the viability and the functional and structural integrity of the cells is preserved. Other factors to be considered are accessibility and cost of the required instrumentation and reagents. For this reason, methods employing spontaneous rosette formation are often more popular than affinity chromatography or cellular immunoabsorbent techniques. Among the latter, nonspecific retention problems and difficulties with the recovery of the depleted population have been noted with some materials. Methods employing antisera plus complement treatment have the disadvantage that the depleted population of cells is destroyed and cannot be recovered. Finally, the problem of modulating cell surface receptors during the separation procedure should be considered. This modulation, although representing an important biological phenomenon, may lead to alteration of some of the functional properties of the cells.

REFERENCES

Ada, G. L., and Byrd, P., 1969, Specific inactivation of antigen-reactive cells with ^{125}I-labelled antigen, *Nature (London)* **222**:1291–1292.
Aiuti, F., Cerottini, J.-C., Coombs, R. R. A., Cooper, M., Dickler, H. B., Frøland, S., Fudenberg, H. H., Greaves, M. F., Grey, H. M., Kunkel, H. G., Natvig, J., Preudhome, J.-L., Rabellino, E., Ritts, R. E., Rowe, D. S., Seligmann, M., Siegal, F. P., Stjernsward, J., Terry, W. D., and Wybran, J., 1974, Special technical report: Identification, enumeration and isolation of B and T lymphocytes from human peripheral blood, *Scand. J. Immunol.* **3**:521–532.
Alexander, E., and Henkart, P., 1976, The adherence of human Fc receptor-bearing lymphocytes to antigen–antibody complexes. II. Morphologic alterations induced by the substrate, *J. Exp. Med.* **143**:329–347.
Alter, B. J., Schendel, D. J., Bach, M. L., Bach, F. H., Klein, J., and Stimpfling, J. H., 1971, Cell mediated lympholysis. Importance of serologically defined H-2 regions, *J. Exp. Med.* **137**:1303–1309.
Altman, A., Cohen, I. R., and Feldman, M., 1973, Normal T cell receptors for alloantigens, *Cell. Immunol.* **7**:134–141.
Ault, K. A., Griffith, A. L., Platsoucas, C. D., and Catsimpoolas, N., 1976, Partial separation of human blood leukocytes by density gradient electrophoresis. Different mobilities of lymphocytes with IgG, those with IgM and IgD, T lymphocytes and monocytes, *J. Immunol.* **117**:1406–1908.
Axelsson, B., Kimura, A., Hammarström, S., Wigzell, H., Nilsson, K., and Mellstedt, H., 1978, *Helix pomatia* A hemagglutinin: Selectivity of binding to lymphocyte surface glycoproteins on T cells and certain B cells, *Eur. J. Immunol.* **8**:757–769.
Bach, J.-F., 1973, Evaluation of T-cells and thymic serum factors in man using the rosette technique, *Transplant. Rev.* **16**:196–217.
Bach, J.-F., Dormont, J., Dardenne, M., and Bolner, H., 1969, *In vitro* rosette inhibition by anti-human anti-lymphocyte serum, *Transplantation* **8**:265–268.
Bach, J.-F., Delvieu, F., and Delbane, F., 1970, The rheumatoid rosette: A diagnostic test unifying seropositive and seronegative rheumatoid arthritis, *Am. J. Med.* **49**:213–222.
Bach, F. H., Segall, M., Stouber-Zier, K., Sondel, P. M., and Alter, B. J., 1973, Cell-mediated

immunity: Separation of cells involved in recognitive and destructive phases, *Science* **180**:403–405.

Barrett, D., 1978, Tissue distribution of human T cells with complement receptors, *Clin. Immunol. Immunopathol.* **11**:190–201.

Basten, A., Sprent, J., and Miller, J. F. A. P., 1972, Receptor for antibody–antigen complexes used to separate T cells from B cells, *Nature (London) (New Biol.)* **235**:178–180.

Baxley, G., Bishop, G. B., Cooper, A. G., and Wortis, H. H., 1973, Rosetting of human red blood cells to thymocytes and thymus-derived cells, *Clin. Exp. Immunol.* **15**:385–392.

Bentwich, Z., Douglas, S. D., Siegal, F. P., and Kunkel, H. G., 1973, Human lymphocyte sheep erythrocyte rosette formation: Some characteristics of the interaction, *Clin. Immunol. Immunopathol.* **1**:511–522.

Berke, G., and Levey, R. H., 1972, Cellular immunoabsorbants in transplantation immunity, *J. Exp. Med.* **135**:972–984.

Bianco, C., 1976, Methods for the study of macrophage Fc and C3 receptors, in *In Vitro Methods in Cell-Mediated and Tumor Immunity* (E. R. Bloom and J. R. David, eds.), pp.407–415, Academic Press, New York.

Bianco, C., and Nussenzweig, V., 1971, Theta-bearing and complement-receptor lymphocytes are distinct population of cells, *Science* **173**:154–156.

Bianco, C., Patrick, R., and Nussenzweig, V., 1970, A population of lymphocytes bearing a membrane receptor for antigen–antibody complement complexes. I. Separation and characterization, *J. Exp. Med.* **132**:702–720.

Binz, H., Lindenmann, J., and Wigzell, H., 1974, Cell-bound receptors for alloantigens on normal lymphocytes, *J. Exp. Med.* **139**:877–893.

Boldt, D. H., MacDermott, R. P., and Jovolan, E. P., 1975, Interaction of plant lectins with purified human lymphocyte populations: Binding characteristics and kinetics of proliferation, *J. Immunol.* **114**:1532–1540.

Boyle, W., 1968, An extension of the ^{51}Cr-release assay for the estimation of mouse cytotoxins, *Transplantation* **6**:761–766.

Boyse, E. A., Old, L. J., and Chomonlinkov, I., 1964, Cytotoxic test for demonstration of mouse antibody, *Methods Med. Res.* **10**:39–47.

Bøyum, A., 1968, Separation of leukocytes from blood and bone marrow, *Scand. J. Clin. Lab. Invest.* **21**(Suppl. 97):9–21.

Braganza, C. M., Stathopoulos, C., Davies, A. J., Elliott, E. V., and Knebel, R. S., 1975, Lymphocyte-erythrocyte (L.E.) rosettes as indicators of the heterogeneity of lymphocytes in a variety of mammalian species, *Cell* **4**:103–106.

Brain, P., Gordon, J., and Willets, W. A., 1970, Rosette formation by peripheral lymphocytes, *Clin. Exp. Immunol.* **6**:681–688.

Brody, T., 1970, Identification of two cell populations required for mouse immunocompetence, *J. Immunol.* **105**:126–135.

Brondz, B. D., 1972, Lymphocyte receptors and mechanisms of *in vitro* cell-mediated immune reactions, *Transplant. Rev.* **10**:112–137.

Brondz, B. D., and Snegiröva, A. E., 1971, Interaction of immune lymphocytes with the mixtures of target cells possessing selected specificities of the H-2 immunizing allele, *Immunology* **20**:457–569.

Brown, C. S., Halpem, H., and Wortis, H. H., 1975, Enhancing rosetting of sheep erythrocytes by human peripheral blood T cells in the presence of Dextran, *Clin. Exp. Immunol.* **20**:505–513.

Burnet, F. M., 1959, *The Clonal Selection Theory of Acquired Immunity*, Cambridge University Press, London.

Byrd, P., and Ada, G. L., 1969, An *in vitro* reaction between labelled flagellin or haemocyanin and lymphocyte-like cells from normal animals, *Immunology* **17**:503–511.

Cantor, H., and Boyse, E. A., 1975, Function subclasses of T lymphocytes bearing different Ly antigens. I. The generation of functionally distinct T-cell subclasses is a differentiative process independent of Ag, *J. Exp. Med.* **141**:1376–1389.

Cantor, H., and Boyse, E. A., 1976, Regulation of cellular and humoral immune responses by T-cell subclasses, *Cold Spring Harbor Symposium,* **XLI**:23–32.

Cantor, H., and Boyse, E., 1977, Regulation of the immune response by T cell subclasses, *Contemp. Top. Immunobiol.* **7**:47–61.

Cantor, H., Shen, F.-W., and Boyse, E. A., 1976, Separation of helper T cells from suppressor T cells expressing different Ly components, *J. Exp. Med.* **143**:1391–1404.

Casali, P., and Perussia, B. M., 1977, C₃-reacted Sepharose: A preparative method for separating T and B lymphocytes, *Clin. Exp. Immunol.* **27**:38–42.

Chapel, H. M., 1973, The effects of papain, thypsin, and phospholipase-A on rosette formation, *Transplantation* **15**:320–331.

Charreire, J., and Bach, J. F., 1974, Self and non-self, *Lancet* **2**:299–300.

Chaves, M. A., and Arranhado, E., 1972, Rosette formation and immunosuppressive agents, *Lancet* **1**:42–43.

Chess, L., and Schlossman, S. F., 1976, Anti-immunoglobulin columns and the separation of T, B and null cells, in *In Vitro Methods in Cell Mediated and Tumor Immunity* (B. R. Bloom and J. R. David, eds.), pp. 255–261, Academic Press, New York.

Chess, L., and Schlossman, S. F., 1977, Human lymphocyte subpopulations, *Adv. Immunol.* **25**:213–241.

Chess, L., MacDermott, R. P., and Schlossman, S. F., 1974a, Immunologic functions of isolated human lymphocyte subpopulations. I. Quantitative isolation of human T and B cells and response to mitogens, *J. Immunol.* **113**:1113–1121.

Chess, L., MacDermott, R. P., and Schlossman, S. F., 1974b, Immunologic functions of isolated human lymphocyte subpopulations. II. Antigen triggering of T and B cells *in vitro, J. Immunol.* **113**:1222–1227.

Chess, L., MacDermott, R. P., Sondel, P., and Schlossman, S., 1974c, Isolation of cells involved in human cellular hypersensitivity, *Prog. Immunol.* **3**:125–132.

Chess, L., Evans, R., Humphreys, R. F., Strominger, J. L., and Schlossman, S. F., 1976, Inhibition of antibody-dependent cellular cytotoxicity and immunoglobulin synthesis by an antiserum prepared against a human B-cell Ia-like molecule. *J. Exp. Med.* **144**:113–122.

Chiao, J. W., and Good, R. A., 1976, Studies of the presence of membrane receptors for complement, IgG and the sheep erythrocyte rosetting capacity on the same human lymphocytes, *Eur J. Immunol.* **6**:157–168.

Chiao, J. W., Pantic, V. S., and Good, R. A., 1974, Human peripheral lymphocytes bearing both B-cell complement receptors and T-cell characteristics for sheep erythrocytes detected by a mixed rosette technique, *Clin. Exp. Immunol.* **18**:483–490.

Chiao, J. W., Pantic, V. S., and Good, R. A., 1975, Human lymphocytes bearing both receptors for complement components and SRBC, *Clin. Immunol. Immunopathol.* **4**:545–552.

Chisholm, P. M., and Ford, W. L., 1978, Selection of antigen-specific cells by adherence to allogeneic cell monolayers: Cytolytic activity, graft-vs-host activity and numbers of adherent and nonadherent cells, *Eur. J. Immunol.* **8**:438–446.

Choi, T. K., Sleight, D. R., and Nisonoff, A., 1974, General method for isolation and recovery of B cells bearing specific receptors, *J. Exp. Med.* **139**:761–766.

Clark, W. R., and Kimura, A. K., 1973, Effect of monolayer fractionation of lymphocytes on graft-vs.-host reactivity, *Transplantation* **16**:110–119.

Cohen, A., and Schlesinger, M., 1970, Absorption of guinea pig serum with agar, *Transplantation* **10**:130–139.

Coombs, R. R. A., Gurner, B. W., Wilson, A. B., Holm, G., and Lindgren, B., 1970, Rosette-formation between human lymphocytes and sheep red cells not involving immunoglobulin receptors, *Int. Arch. Allergy Appl. Immunol.* **39:**658–672.

Cordier, G., Samarut, C., and Revillard, J. P., 1977, Changes of Fcγ receptor-related properties induced by interaction of human lymphocytes with insoluble immune complexes, *J. Immunol.* **119:**1943–1949.

Davidson, W. F., and Parish, C. R., 1975, A procedure for removing red cells and dead cells from lymphoid cell suspensions, *J. Immunol. Methods* **7:**291–300.

Dickler, H. B., and Kunkel, H. G., 1972, Interaction of aggregated gammaglobulin with B-lymphocytes, *J. Exp. Med.* **136:**191–196.

Dickler, H. B., Adkinson, M. F., and Terry, W. D., 1974, Evidence for individual human peripheral blood lymphocytes bearing both B and T cell markers, *Nature* **247:**213–215.

Dierich, M. P., Pellegrino, M. A., Ferrone, S., and Reisfeld, R. A., 1974, Evaluation of C_3 receptors on lymphoid cells with different complement sources, *J. Immunol.* **112:**1766–1772.

Djeu, J., Payne, S., Alford, C., Heim, W., Pomeroy, T., Cohen, M., Oldham, R., and Herberman, R. B., 1977, Detection of decreased proportion of lymphocytes forming rosettes with sheep erythrocytes at 29°C in the blood of cancer patients, *Clin. Immunol. Immunopathol.* **8:**405–411.

Djordjevic, B., and Szybalski, W., 1960, Genetics of human cell lines, *J. Exp. Med.* **112:**509–521.

Dorval, G., Wolsh, K. I., Wigzell, H., 1974, Labeled staphylococcal protein A as an immunological probe in the analysis of cell surface markers, *Scand. J. Immunol.* **3:**405–414.

Dwyer, J. M., 1976, Identifying and enumerating human T and B lymphocytes, *Prog. Allergy* **21:**178–191.

Edelman, G. M., Rutishauser, V., and Millette, C. F., 1971, Cell fractionation and arrangement on fibers, beads, and surfaces, *Proc. Natl. Acad. Sci. USA* **68:**2153–2158.

Ehlenberger, A. G., and Nussenzweig, V., 1976, Identification of cells with complement receptors, in *In Vitro Methods in Cell-Mediated and Tumor Immunity* (E. R. Bloom and J. R. David, eds.), pp. 113–121, Academic Press, New York.

Ferrarini, M., Moretta, L., Abrile, R., and Durante, M. L., 1975, Receptors for IgG molecules on human lymphocytes forming spontaneous rosettes with sheep red cells, *Eur. J. Immunol.* **5:**70–72.

Florey, M. J., and Peetoom, F., 1976, Modified E-rosette test for detection of total and active rosette forming lymphocytes, *J. Immunol. Methods* **13:**201–208.

Fournier, C., and Charreire, J., 1978, Activation of a human T cell subpopulation bearing receptors for autologous erythrocytes by concanavalin A, *J. Immunol.* **121:**771.-779.

Frøland, S. S., 1972, Binding of sheep erythrocytes to human lymphocytes. A probable marker of T lymphocytes, *Scand. J. Immunol.* **1:**269–276.

Frøland, S., and Natvig, J. B., 1973, Identification of three different human lymphocyte populations by surface markers, *Transplant. Rev.* **16:**114–169.

Frøland, S., Wisloff, F., and Michaelson, T. E., 1974, Human lymphocytes with receptors for IgG, a population of cells distinct from T and B lymphocytes, *Inter. Arch. Allergy Appl. Immunol.* **47:**124–138.

Frøland, S. S., and Wisloff, F., 1976, A rosette technique for identification of human lymphocytes with Fc receptors, in *In Vitro Methods in Cell-Mediated and Tumor Immunity* (B. R. Bloom and J. R. David, eds.), pp. 137–142, Academic Press, New York.

Galili, U., and Schlesinger, M., 1975, Subpopulations of human thymus cells differing in their capacity to form stable E-rosettes and in their immunologic reactivity, *J. Immunol.* **115:**827–833.

Gelfand, M. C., Shin, M. L., Nagle, R. B., Green, I., and Frank, M. M., 1976, The glomerular complement receptor in immunologically mediated renal glomerular injury, *N. Engl. J. Med.* **295**:10–14.

Ghetie, V., Nilsson, K., and Sjöquist, J., 1974, Density gradient separation of lymphoid cells adhering to protein A containing staphylococci, *Proc. Natl. Acad. Sci. USA* **71**:4831–4835.

Ghetie, V., Stalenheim, G., and Sjöquist, J., 1975, Cell separation by staphylococcal protein A-coated erythrocytes, *Scand. J. Immunol.* **4**:471–477.

Ghetie, V., Mota, G., and Sjöquist, J., 1978, Separation of cells by affinity chromatography on SpA-sepharose 6MB, *J. Immunol. Methods* **21**:133–141.

Gilbertsen, R. B., and Metzgar, R. S., 1976, Human T and B lymphocyte rosette tests: Effect of enzymatic modification of sheep erythrocytes (E) and the specificity of neuraminidase-treated E, *Cell. Immunol.* **24**:97–106.

Ginsburg, H., Ax, W., and Berke, G., 1969, Graft reaction in tissue culture by normal rat lymphocytes, *Transplant. Proc.* **1**:551–582.

Giuliano, V. J., Jasin, H. E., Hurd, E. R., and Ziff, M., 1974, Enumeration of B-lymphocytes in human peripheral blood by a rosette method for the detection of surface-bound immunoglobulin, *J. Immunol.* **112**:1494–1499.

Gluckman, J. C., and Motnambault, P., 1975, Spontaneous autorosette-forming cells in man: A marker for a subset population of T-lymphocytes? *Clin. Exp. Immunol.* **22**:302–310.

Gmelig-Meyling, F. H. J., Keoy-Blok, L., and Ballieux, R. E., 1974, Complement-dependent cytolysis of human B lymphocytes with anti-light chain antisera, *Eur. J. Immunol.* **4**:332–337.

Gmelig-Meyling, F., Van Der Harn, M., and Ballieux, R. E., 1976, Binding of IgM by human T lymphocytes, *Scand. J. Immunol.* **5**:487–493.

Golan, D. T., and Borel, Y., 1972, Detection of hapten-binding cells by a highly radioactive ^{125}I-conjugate, *J. Exp. Med.* **136**:305–317.

Gold, E. R., and Fudenberg, H. H., 1967, Chromic chloride: A coupling reagent for passive hemagglutination reactions, *J. Immunol.* **99**:859–966.

Goldstein, I. J., Hammarström, S., and Sundbland, G., 1975, Precipitation and carbohydrate-binding specificity studies on wheat germ agglutinin, *Biochim. Biophys. Acta* **405**:53–65.

Goldstein, P., Svedmyr, E., and Wigzell, H., 1971, Cells mediating specific *in vitro* cytotoxicity, *J. Exp. Med.* **134**:1385–1397.

Good, R. A., 1972, Recent studies on the immunodeficiencies of man, *Am. J. Pathol.* **69**:489–490.

Greaves, M. F., and Brown, G., 1974, Purification of human T and B lymphocytes. *J. Immunol.* **112**:420–429.

Griffin, F. M., Bianco, C., and Silverstein, S. C., 1975, Characterization of the macrophage receptor for complement and demonstration of its functional independence from the receptor for the Fc portion of immunoglobulin G, *J. Exp. Med.* **141**:1269–1282.

Gross, R. L., Latty, S., Williams, E. L., and Newberne, P. M., 1975, Abnormal spontaneous rosette formation and rosette inhibition in lung carcinoma, *N. Engl. J. Med.* **292**:439–443.

Gupta, S, and Good, R. A., 1978, Human T cell subsets in health and disease, in *Human Lymphocyte Differentiation: Its Application to Human Cancer* (C. B. Serrou and C. Rosenfeld, eds.), pp. 367–375, Elsevier North-Holland Biomedical Press, Amsterdam.

Gupta, S., and Grieco, M. H., 1974, E-rosette test, *Lancet* **2**:954–955.

Gupta, S., and Grieco, M. H., 1975, Rosette formation with mouse erythrocytes—probable marker for human B lymphocytes, *Inter. Arch. Allergy Appl. Immunol.* **49**:734–742.

Gupta, S., Good, R. A., and Siegal, F. P., 1976a, Rosette formation with mouse erythrocytes. III. Studies in patients with primary immunodeficiency and lymphoproliferative disorders, *Clin. Exp. Immunol.* **25**:319–327.

Gupta, S., Ross, G., Good, R. A., and Siegal, F. P., 1976b, Surface markers on human eosinophils, *Blood* **48**:755–793.

Gupta, S., Fernandes, G., Nair, M., and Good, R. A., 1978, Spontaneous and antibody-dependent cell cytotoxicity by human T cell subpopulation, *Proc. Natl. Acad. Sci. USA* **75**:5137–5141.

Haas, W., 1975, Separation of antigen-specific lymphocytes. II. Enrichment of hapten-specific antibody-forming cell precursor, *J. Exp. Med.* **141**:1015–1029.

Haas, W., and Layton, J. E., 1975, Separation of antigen-specific lymphocytes. I. Enrichment of antigen-binding cells, *J. Exp. Med.* **141**:1004–1014.

Haas, W., Schrader, J. W., and Szenberg, A., 1974, A new simple method for the preparation of lymphocytes bearing specific receptors, *Eur. J. Immunol.* **4**:565–601.

Hallberg, T., Burner, B. W., and Coombs, R. R. A., 1973, Opsonic adherence of sensitized ox red cells to human lymphocytes as measured by rosette formation, *Inter. Arch. Allergy Appl. Immunol.* **44**:500–513.

Haller, O., Gidlund, M., Hellström, U., Hammarström, S., and Wigzell, H., 1978, A new surface marker on mouse natural killer cells: Receptors for *Helix pomatia* A hemagglutinin, *Eur. J. Immunol.* **8**:765–771.

Hammarström, S., Hellström, U., Perlmann, P., and Dillner, M. L., 1973, A new surface marker on T lymphocytes of human peripheral blood, *J. Exp. Med.* **138**:1270–1275.

Häyry, P., Anderson, L. C., Gahmberg, C., Roberts, P., Ranki, A., Nordling, S., 1975, Fractionation of immunocompetent cells by free-flow cell electrophoresis, *Israel J. Med. Sci.* **11**:1299–1318.

Heier, H. E., 1974, The influence of mechanical force on the rosette test for human T lymphocytes, *Scand. J. Immunol.* **3**:677–700.

Hellström, U., Hammarström, S., Dillner, M. L., Perlmann, H., and Perlmann, P., 1976, Fractionation of human blood lymphocytes on *Helix pomatia* A haemagglutinin coupled to Sepharose beads. *Scand. J. Immunol.* **5**(*Suppl.* 5):45–62.

Hoffman, T., and Kunkel, H. G., 1976, The E rosette test, in *In Vitro Methods in Cell-Mediated and Tumor Immunity* (B. R. Bloom and J. R. David, eds.), pp. 71–81, Academic Press, New York.

Horowitz, D. A., and Lobo, D. I., 1975, Characterization of two populations of human lymphocytes bearing easily detectable surface immunoglobulin, *J. Clin. Invest.* **56**:1464–1472.

Hsu, C. C. S., and Fell, A., 1974, Polymorphonuclear cells form E rosettes, *N. Engl. J. Med.* **290**:402–403.

Huber, A., Douglas, S. D., and Fudenberg, H. H., 1969, The IgA receptor: An immunological marker for the characterization of mononuclear cells, *Immunology* **17**:7–21.

Johnson, A. H., Scott, D. W., McKeown, P. T., Pool, P. A., and Amos, D. B., 1977, Affinity chromatography with antifluorescein antibody to separate Ig-positive cells: Preliminary report. *Transplant Proc.* **9**(*Suppl.* 1):145–148.

Johnson, J., 1977, *Annual Report of the Basel Institute of Immunology, Communication 1201.*

Jondal, M., 1976a, SRBC rosette formation as a human T lymphocyte marker, *Scand. J. Immunol.* **5** (*Suppl.* 5): 69–76.

Jondal, M., 1976b, Spontaneous lymphocyte-mediated cytotoxicity (SLMC), in *In Vitro Methods of Cell-Mediated and Tumor Immunity* (B. R. Bloom and J. R. David, eds.), pp. 263–266, Academic Press, New York.

Jondal, M., Holm, G., and Wigzell, H., 1972, Surface markers on human B and T lymphocytes. I. A large population of lymphocytes forming non-immune rosettes with sheep red blood cells, *J. Exp. Med.* **136**:207–215.

Jondal, M., Wigzell, H., and Aiuti, F., 1973, Human lymphocyte subpopulations. Classification according to surface markers and/or functional characteristics, *Transplant. Rev.* **16**:163–216.

Julius, M. H., and Herzenberg, L. A., 1974, Isolation of antigen-binding cells from unprimed mice, *J. Exp. Med.* **140**:904–913.

Julius, M. H., Masuda, T., Herzenberg, L. A., 1972, Demonstration that antigen-binding cells are precursors of antibody producing cells after purification with a fluorescence activated cell sorter, *Proc. Natl. Acad. Sci. USA* **69**:1934–1939.

Kaplan, J., 1975, Human T lymphocytes form rosettes with autologous and allogeneic human red blood cells, *Clin. Immunol. Immunopathol.* **3**:471–475.

Kaplan, M. E., and Clark, C. J., 1974, An improved rosetting assay for detection of human T lymphocytes, *J. Immunol. Methods* **5**:131–137.

Kaplan, M. E., Woodson, M., and Clark, C., 1976, Detection of human T lymphocytes by rosette formation with AET-treated sheep red cells, in *In Vitro Methods in Cell-Mediated and Tumor Immunity* (B. R. Bloom and J. R. David, eds.), pp. 83–88, Academic Press, New York.

Karpf, M., Gelfand, M. C., Handwenger, B. S., and Schwartz, R. H., 1975, Lack of B lymphocyte depletion from murine spleen cell populations by a human γ-globulin column system, *J. Immunol.* **114**:542–549.

Karsenti, E., Bomens, M. and Avrameas, S., 1975, Stimulation and inhibition of DNA synthesis in rat thymocytes: Action of concanavalin A and wheat germ agglutinin, *Eur. J. Immunol.* **5**:74–81.

Katz, D. H., and Benacerraff, B., 1972, The regulatory influence of activated T cells on B cell responses to antigen, *Adv. Immunol.* **15**:1–27.

Kay, H. D., Bonnard, G. D., West, W. H., Herberman, R. B., 1977, A functional comparison of human Fc-receptor-bearing lymphocytes active in natural cytotoxicity and antibody-dependent cellular cytotoxicity, *J. Immunol.* **118**: 2058–2066.

Kedar, E., Ortiz de Landazuri, M., and Bonavida, B., 1974, Cellular immunoabsorbents: A simplified technique for separation of lymphoid cell populations, *J. Immunol.* **112**:1231–1243.

Kennedy, J. C. and Axelrad, M. A., 1971, An improved assay for haemolytic plaque-forming cells, *Immunology* **20**:253–258.

Kofler, R., and Wick, G., 1977, Some methodological aspects of the chromium chloride method for coupling antigen to erythrocytes, *J. Immunol. Methods* **16**:201–209.

Kondorosi, E., Nagy, J., and Dénes, G., 1977, Optimal conditions for the separation of rat lymphocytes on anti-immunoglobulin–immunoglobulin affinity columns, *J. Immunol. Methods* **16**:1–13.

Kurnick, J. T., and Grey, H. M., 1975, Relationship between immunoglobulin-bearing lymphocytes and cells reactive with sensitized human erythrocytes, *J. Immunol.* **115**:305–307.

Lay, W. H., Mendes, N. F., Bianco, C., and Nussenzweig, V., 1971, Binding of sheep red blood cells to a large population of human lymphocytes, *Nature (London)* **230**:531–532.

Ling, N. R., Bishop, S., and Jeffries, R., 1977, Use of antibody-coated red cells for the sensitive detection of antigen and in rosette tests for cells bearing surface immunoglobulins, *J. Immunol. Methods* **15**:279–286.

Lobo, P. I., Westervelt, F. B., and Horowitz, D. A., 1975, Identification of two populations of immunoglobulin bearing lymphocytes in man. *J. Immunol.* **114**:116–121.

Lohrmann, H. P., and Novikous, L., 1974, Rosette formation between T-lymphocytes and unsensitized rhesus monkey erythrocytes, *Clin. Immunol. Immunopathol.***3**:99–111.

Lonai, P., Eliraz, A., Wekerle, H., and Feldman, M., 1973, Depletion of specific graft-versus-host reactivity following absorption of nonsensitized lymphocytes on allogeneic fibroblasts, *Transplantation* **15**:368–393.

London, J., Berrich, S., and Bach, J. -F., 1978, Peanut agglutinin—a new tool for studying T lymphocyte subpopulations, *J. Immunol.* **121**:438–497.

Lotan, R., Skutelsky, E., Damon, D., and Sharon, N., 1975, The purification composition, and specificity of the anti-T lectin from peanut (*Arachis hypogaea*), *J. Biol. Chem.* **250:**8518–8529.

MacDermott, R. P., Chess, L., and Schlossman, S. F., 1975, Immunologic functions of isolated human lymphocyte subpopulations, *Clin. Immunol. Immunopathol.* **4:**415–422.

Mage, M G., and McHugh, L. L., 1973, Retention of graft vs. host activity in non-adherent spleen cells after depletion of cytotoxic activity by incubation on allogeneic target cells, *J. Immunol.* **111:**652–660.

Mage, M. G., and McHugh, L. L., 1975, Specific partial depletion of graft vs. host activity by incubation and centrifugation of mouse spleen cells on allogeneic spleen cell monolayers, *J. Immunol.* **115:**911–922.

Mage, M. G., McHugh, L. L., and Rothstein, T. L., 1977, Mouse lymphocytes with and without surface immunoglobulin: Preparative scale separation in polystyrene tissue culture dishes coated with specifically purified anti-immunoglobulin, *J. Immunol. Methods* **15:**47–56.

McArthur, W. P., Chapman, J., and Thorbecke, G. J., 1971, Immunocompetent cells of the chicken, *J. Exp. Med.* **134:**1036–1047.

Mendes, N. F., Tolmai, M. E. A., Selveira, N. P. A., Gilbertson, R. B., and Metzgar, R. S., 1973, Technical aspects of the rosette tests used to detect human complement receptor (B) and sheep erythrocyte-binding (T) lymphocytes, *J. Immunol.* **111:**860–868.

Mendes, N. F., Miki, S. S., and Peixinho, F., 1974, Combined detection of human T and B lymphocytes by rosette formation with sheep erythrocytes and Zynosan C₃ complexes, *J. Immunol.* **113:**531–537.

Miller, G. W., Saluk, P. H., and Nussenzweig, V., 1973, Complement-dependent release of immune complexes from the lymphocyte membrane, *J. Exp. Med.* **138:**495–597.

Miller, J. F. A. P., and Mitchell, G. F., 1969, Thymus and antigen-reactive cells, *Transplant. Rev.* **1:**3–42.

Miller, J. F. A. P., Sprent, J., Basten, A., and Warner, N. L., 1972, Selective cytotoxicity of anti-kappa serum for B lymphocytes, *Nature (London) (New Biol.)* **237:**18–20.

Moretta, L., Ferrarini, M., Durante, M. L., and Mingari, M. C., 1975, Expression of a receptor for IgM by human T cells *in vitro, Euro. J. Immunol.* **5:**565–570.

Moretta, L., Ferrarini, M., Mingari, M. C., Moretta, A., and Webb, S. R., 1976a, Subpopulations of human T cells identified by receptor for immunoglobulins and mitogen responsiveness, *J. Immunol.* **117:**2171–2177.

Moretta, L., Mingari, M. C., and Romanzi, C. A., 1976b, Loss of Fc receptors for IgG from human T lymphocytes exposed to IgG immune complexes, *Nature (London)* **272:**618–620.

Moretta, L., Webb, S. R., Rossi, C. E., Lydyard, P. M., and Cooper, M. D., 1977, Functional analysis of two subpopulations of human T cells and their distribution in immunodeficient patients, *J. Exp. Med.* **146:**184–197.

Moretta, L., Ferrarini, M., and Cooper, M. D., 1978, Characterization of human T-cell subpopulations as defined by specific receptors for immunoglobulin, in *Contemporary Topics in Immunobiology* (N. L. Warner and M. D. Cooper, eds.), Volume 8, pp. 19–53, Plenum, New York.

Murphy, D. B., Herzenberg, L. A., Okumura, K., Herzenberg, L. A., and McDevitt, H. O., 1976, A new I subregion (I-J) marked by a locus (Ia-4) controlling surface determinants on suppressor T-lymphocytes, *J. Exp. Med.* **144:**699–708.

Nagata, Y., and Burger, M. M., 1974, Wheat germ agglutinin. Molecular characteristics and specificity for sugar binding, *J. Biol. Chem.* **249:**3116–3122.

Naor, E., and Sulitzean, P., 1967, Binding of radioiodinated bovine serum albumin to mouse spleen cells, *Nature (London)* **214:**687–689.

Natvig, J. B., and Frøland, S. S., 1976, Detection of a third lymphocyte-like cell type by rosette formation with erythrocytes sensitized by various anti-Rh antibodies, *Scand. J. Immunol.* **5**(*Suppl.* 5):83–89.

Neefe, J. R., and Sachs, D. H., 1976, Specific elimination of cytotoxic effector cells, *J. Exp. Med.* **144**:996–1006.

Nossal, G. J. V., and Pike, B. L., 1976, Single cell studies on the antibody-forming potential of fractionated, hapten-specific B lymphocytes, *Immunology* **30**:189–191.

Nossal, G. J. V., and Pike, B. L., 1978, Improved procedures for the fractionation and *in vitro* stimulation of hapten-specific B lymphocytes, *J. Immunol.* **120**:145–150.

Nossal, G. J. V., Pike, B. L., and Battye, F. L., 1978, Sequential use of hapten-gelatin fractionation and fluorescence-activated cell sorting in the enrichment of hapten-specific B lymphocytes, *Eur. J. Immunol.* **8**:151–157.

Okumura, K., Takemori, T., Tokuhisa, T., and Tada, T., 1977, Specific enrichment of the suppressor T cell bearing I-J determinants. Parallel functional and serological characterizations, *J. Exp. Med.* **146**:1234–1245.

Osoba, D., 1970, Some physical and radiobiological properties of immunologically reactive mouse spleen cells, *J. Exp. Med.* **132**:368–382.

Parish, C. R., 1975, Separation and functional analysis of subpopulations of lymphocytes bearing complement and Fc receptors, *Transplant Rev.* **25**:98–120.

Parish, C. R., and Hayward, J. A., 1974a, The lymphocyte surface. I. Relation between Fc receptors, C_3 receptors and surface immunoglobulin. *Proc. R. Soc. London Ser. B* **187**:47–63.

Parish, C. R., and Hayward, J. A., 1974b, The lymphocyte surface. II. Separation of Fc receptor, C_3 receptor and surface immunoglobulin-bearing lymphocytes, *Proc. R. Soc. London Ser. B* **187**:65–81.

Parish, C. R., and Hayward, J. A., 1974c, The lymphocyte surface. III. Function of Fc receptor, C_3 receptor and surface Ig bearing lymphocytes: Identification of a radioresistant B cell, *Proc. R. Soc. London Ser. B* **187**:379–395.

Parish, C. R., and McKenzie, I. F. C., 1977, Direct visualization of T lymphocytes bearing Ia antigens controlled by the I-J subregion, *J. Exp. Med.* **146**:332–362.

Parish, C. R., and McKenzie, I. F. C., 1978, A sensitive rosetting method for detecting subpopulations of lymphocytes which react with alloantisera, *J. Immunol. Methods* **20**:173–183.

Parish, C. R., Kirov, S. M., Bowen, N., and Blanden, R. V., 1974, A one-step procedure for separating mouse T and B lymphocytes, *Eur. J. Immunol.* **4**:808–815.

Patel, P. C., Menezes, J., Bourkas, A., Dorval, G., Rivard, G. E., Boulay, G., Stanley, P., and Joncas, J. H., 1978, Rosette formation by human lymphoid cells with monkey red blood cells, *Ann. Immunol. (Paris)* **120c**:449–552.

Pellegrino, M. A., Ferrone, S., Dierich, M. P., and Reisfeld, R. A., 1975a, Enhancement of sheep red blood cell human lymphocyte-rosette formation by the sulfhydryl compound 2-amino ethylisothiouronium bromide, *Clin. Immunol. Immunopathol.* **3**:324–331.

Pellegrino, M. A., Ferrone, S., and Theofilopoulos, A. N., 1975b, Rosette formation of human lymphoid cells with monkey red blood cells, *J. Immunol.* **115**:1065–1071.

Pellegrino, M. A., Ferrone, S., and Theofilopoulos, A. N., 1976, Isolation of human T and B lymphocytes by rosette formation with 2 aminoethylisothiouronium bromide (AET)-treated sheep red blood cells and with monkey red blood cells, *J. Immunol. Methods* **11**:273–279.

Perlmann, P., Perlmann, H., and Wigzell, H., 1972, Lymphocyte mediated cytotoxicity *in vitro*. Induction and inhibition by humoral antibody and nature of effector cells, *Transplant. Rev.* **13**:91–114.

Perlmann, P., Wigzell, H., Goldstein, P., Laruan, E. W., Larsson, A., O'Toole, C., Perlmann, H., and Svedmyr, E. A. J., 1973, Cell-mediated cytolysis *in vitro*: Analysis of active lymphocyte subpopulations in different experimental systems, *Adv. Biosci.* **21**:71–97.

Perlmann, H., Perlmann, P., Pape, G. R., and Hallden, G., 1976, Purification, fractionation and assay of antibody-dependent lymphocytic effector K cells in human blood, *Scand. J. Immunol.* **5**(*Suppl.* 5):57–68.

Pichler, W. J., and Knapp. W., 1978, Receptors for IgM on human B lymphocytes, *Scand. J. Immunol.* **1**:105–109.

Platsoucas, C. D., Good, R. A., and Gupta, S., 1979, Separation of human T lymphocyte subpopulations (Tμ, Tγ) by density gradient electrophoresis, *Proc. Natl. Acad. Sci. USA* **76**:1972–1976.

Potash, M. J., and Knopf, P. M., 1978, Differential sensitivity of memory cell subpopulations to anti-immunoglubulin and complement, *Eur. J. Immunol.* **8**:711–715.

Press, J. L., Klinman, R. R., and McDevitt, H. O., 1976, Expression of Ia antigens on hapten-specific B cells, *J. Exp. Med.* **144**:414–426.

Puck, T. T., and Kao, F., 1967, Genetics of somatic mammalian cells. V. Treatment with 5-bromodeoxyuridine and usable light for isolation of nutritionally deficient mutants, *Proc. Natl. Acad. Sci. USA* **58**:1227–1321.

Rabellino, E. M., and Metcalf, D., 1975, Receptors for C_3 and IgG on macrophage neutrophil and eosinophil colony cells grown *in vitro*, *J. Immunol.* **115**:688–727.

Raff, M. C., 1970, Role of thymus-derived lymphocytes in the secondary humoral immune response in mice, *Nature (London)* **226**:1257–1258.

Reisner, Y., Linker-Israel, M., and Sharon, N., 1976a, Separation of mouse thymocytes into two subpopulations by the use of peanut lectin, *Cell. Immunol.* **25**:129–137.

Reisner, Y., Ravid, A., and Sharon, N., 1976b, Use of soybean agglutinin for the separation of mouse B and T lymphocytes, *Biochem. Biophys. Res. Commun.* **72**:1585–1591.

Reisner, Y., Hzicoviter, L., Meshrer, A., and Sharon, N., 1978, Hemopoietic stem cell transplantation using mouse bone marrow and spleen cells fractionated by lectins, *Proc. Natl. Acad. Sci. USA* **75**:2933–2937.

Roelants, G. E., and Askonas, B. A., 1971, Cell cooperation in antibody induction. The susceptibility of helper cells to specific lethal radioactive antigen, *Eur. J. Immunol.* **1**:151–159.

Ross, G. D., and Polley, M. J., 1975, Specificity of human lymphocyte complement receptors, *J. Exp. Med.* **141**:1163–1180.

Ross, G. D., and Polley, M. J., 1976, Detection of complement-receptor lymphocytes (CRL), in *In Vitro Methods in Cell-Mediated and Tumor Immunity* (E. R. Bloom and J. R. David, eds.), pp. 123–136, Academic Press, New York.

Ross, G. D., Polley, M. J., Rabellino, E. M., and Grey, H. M., 1973, Two different complement receptors on human lymphocytes, *J. Exp. Med.* **138**:798–814.

Ross, G. D., Rabellino, E. M., and Polley, M. J., 1976, Mouse leukocyte C_3 receptors, *Fed. Proc.* **35**:254.

Rubin, B., 1975, Studies on the absorbability of graft vs. host reactive lymphocytes, *Clin. Exp. Immunol.* **20**:513–519.

Ryser, J.-E., and Vassali, P., 1974, Mouse bone marrow lymphocytes and their differentiation, *J. Immunol.* **113**:719–726.

Sandilands, G. P., Gray, K. G., Cooney, A. E., Browning, J. D., and Anderson, J. R., 1974, Auto-rosette formation by human thymocytes and lymphocytes, *Lancet* **1**:27–28.

Sandrin, M. S., Potter, T. A., Morgan, G. M., and McKenzie, I. F. C., 1978, Detection of mouse alloantibodies by rosetting with protein A-coated sheep red blood cells, *Transplantation* **26**:126–129.

Samarut, C., Drochier, J., and Revillard, J. P., 1976, Distribution of cells binding erythrocyte-antibody (EA) complexes in human lymphoid populations, *Scand. J. Immunol.* **5**:221–227.

Saxon, A., Feldhaus, J., and Robins, R. A., 1976, Single step separation of human T and B cells using AET treated SRBC rosettes, *J. Immunol. Methods* **12:**285–292.

Scher, I., Sharrow, S. O., Wistar, R., Jr., Asofsky, R., and Paul, W. E., 1976, B-lymphocyte heterogeneity: Ontogenetic development and organ distribution of B-lymphocyte populations defined by their density of surface immunoglobulin, *J. Exp. Med.* **144:**494–509.

Schlossman, S. F., and Hudson, L., 1973, Specific purification of lymphocytes populations on a digestible immunoabsorbent, *J. Immunol.* **110:**313–315.

Scott, D. W., 1976a, Cellular events in tolerance vs. detection, isolation, and fate of lymphoid cells which bind fluorosceinated antigens *in vivo, Cell. Immunol.* **22:**311–413.

Scott, D. W., 1976b, Antifluorescein affinity columns isolation and immunocompetence of lymphocytes that bind fluoresceinated antigens *in vivo* or *in vitro, J. Exp. Med.* **144:**69–78.

Seaman, G. V. F., and Uhlenbruck, G., 1963, The surface of erythrocytes from some animal sources, *Arch. Biochem. Biophys.* **100:**493–502.

Shortman, K., Williams, N., and Adams, P., 1972, The separation of different cell classes from lymphoid organs. V. Simple procedures for the removal of cell debris, damaged cells and erythroid cells from lymphoid suspensions, *J. Immunol. Methods* **1:**273–278.

Singer, K. H., Johnston, C., Amos, D. B., and Scott, D. W., 1978, Selective depletion and enrichment of alloreactive cytolytic effector lymphocytes using anti-fluorescein affinity columns, *Cell Immunol.* **36:**75–85.

Smith, R. A., Kerman, R., Ezdinli, E., and Stefani, S., 1975, A modified assay for the detection of human adult active rosette forming lymphocytes, *J. Immunol. Methods* **8:**175–181.

Stathopoulos, G., and Elliot, E. V., 1974, Formation of mouse or sheep red blood cell rosettes by lymphocytes from normal and leukemic individuals, *Lancet* **2:**600–602.

Steel, C. M., Evans, J., Smith, M. A., 1975, The sheep-cell rosette test on human peripheral blood lymphocytes: An analysis of some variable factors in the technique, *Brit. J. Haematol.* **28:**245–252.

Stout, R. D., and Herzenberg, L. A., 1975, The Fc receptor on thymus derived lymphocytes. II. Mitogen responsiveness of T lymphocytes bearing the Fc receptor, *J. Exp. Med.* **142:**1041–1050.

Strelkauskas, A. J., Teodorescu, M., and Dray, S., 1975, Enumeration and isolation of human T and B lymphocytes by rosette formation with antibody-coated erythrocytes, *Clin. Exp. Immunol.* **22:**62–67.

Strelkauskas, A. J., Schaut, V., Wilson, B. S., Chess, L., and Schlossman, S. F., 1978, Isolation and characterization of naturally occurring subclasses of human peripheral blood T cells with regulatory functions, *J. Immunol.* **120:**1278–1286.

Stulting, D., and Berke, G., 1973, Nature of lymphocyte-tumor interaction, A general method for cellular immunoabsorption, *J. Exp. Med.* **137:**932–945.

Stulting, R. D., and Berke, G., 1974, Cellular immunoabsorbents. A new approach in transplantation and tumor immunology, *Israel J. Med. Sci.* **10:**992–1000.

Takahashi, T., Old, L. J., McIntire, R., and Boyse, E. A., 1971, Immunoglobulin and other surface antigens of cells of the immune system, *J. Exp. Med.* **134:**815–824.

Taniguchi, M., and Miller, J. F. A. P., 1977, Enrichment of specific suppressor T cells and characterizations of their surface markers, *J. Exp. Med.* **146:**1450–1459.

Taniguchi, N., Okuda, N., Moriya, N., Miyawaki, T., and Nagaski, T., 1976, Inhibitory effect of sheep erythrocyte fragments on rosette formation of human T lymphocytes with sheep red blood cells, *Clin. Exp. Immunol.* **24:**370–373.

Targan, S., and Jondal, M., 1978, Monolayer immune complex (MIC) fractionation of Fc receptor bearing human spontaneous killer cells, *J. Immunol. Methods* **22:**123–129.

Theofilopoulos, A. N., Bokisch, V. A., and Dixon, F. J., 1974, Receptor for soluble C_3 and C_3b on human lymphoblastoid (Raji) cells, *J. Exp. Med.* **139:**696–704.

Tönder, O., Morse, P. A., and Humphrey, L. J., 1974, Similarities of Fc receptors in human malignant tissue and normal lymphoid tissue, *J. Immunol.* **113**:1162–1169.

Truffa-Bachi, P., and Wofsy, L., 1970, Specific separation of cells on affinity columns, *Proc. Natl. Acad. Sci. USA* **66**:685–689.

Uhlenbruck, G., Seaman, G. V. F., Coombs, R. R. A., 1967, Factors influencing the agglutinability of red cells. III. Physico-chemical studies on ox red cells of different classes of agglutinability, *Vox Sang.* **12**:420–428.

Van Boxel, J., and Rosenstreich, D. L., 1974, Binding of aggregated γ-globulin to activated T lymphocytes in guinea pig, *J. Exp. Med.* **139**:1002–1014.

von Boehmer, H., and Shortman, K., 1973, The separation of different cell classes from lymphoid organs. IX. A simple and rapid method for removal of damaged cells from lymphoid cell suspensions, *J. Immunol. Methods* **2**:293–301.

Wahl, S. J., Everson, G. M., and Oppenheim, J., 1974, Induction of guinea pig B cell lymphokine synthesis by mitogenic and non-mitogenic signals to Fc, Ig, and C_3 receptors, *J. Exp. Med.* **140**:1631–1644.

Wahl, S. M., Rosenstreich, D. L., and Oppenheim, J. J., 1976, Separation of human lymphocytes by E rosette sedimentation, in *In Vitro Methods in Cell-Mediated and Tumor Immunity* (B. R. Bloom and J. R. David, eds.), pp. 231–240, Academic Press, New York.

Webb, S. R., and Cooper, M. D., 1973, T cells can bind antigen via cytophilic IgM antibody, made by B cells, *J. Immunol.* **111**:275–281.

Weiner, M. S., Bianco, C., and Nussenzweig, V., 1973, Enhanced binding of neuraminidase-treated sheep erythrocytes to human T lymphocytes, *Blood* **42**:939–951.

West, W. H., Sienknecht, C. W., Townes, A. S., and Herberman, R. B., 1976, Performance of a rosette assay between lymphocytes and sheep erythrocytes at elevated temperatures to study patients with cancer and other diseases, *Clin. Immunol. Immunopathol.* **5**:60–66.

West, W. H., Cannon, G. B., Kay, H. D., Bonnard, G. D., and Herberman, R. B., 1977a, Natural cytotoxic reactivity of human lymphocytes against a myeloid cell line: Characterization of effector cells, *J. Immunol.* **118**:355–36l.

West, W. H., Payne, S. M., Weese, J. L., and Herberman, R. B., 1977b, Human T lymphocyte subpopulations: Correlation between E-rosette-forming affinity and expression of the Fc receptor, *J. Immunol.* **119**:548–553.

West, W. H., Boozer, R. B., and Herberman, R. B., 1978, Low affinity E-rosette formation by the human K cell, *J. Immunol.* **120**:90–95.

Wigzell, H., 1970, Specific fractionation of immunocompetent cells, *Transplant. Rev.* **5**:76–96.

Wigzell, H., 1971, Cellular immunoabsorbents, in *Progress in Immunology* (B. Amos, ed.), Academic Press, pp. 1105–1113, New York.

Wigzell, H., 1976a, Enrichment or depletion of surface-immunoglobulin-coated cells using anti-immunoglobulin antibodies and glass or plastic bead columns, in *In Vitro Methods in Cell-Mediated and Tumor Immunity* (B. R. Bloom and J. R. David, eds.), pp. 245–253, Academic Press, New York.

Wigzell, H., 1976b, Specific affinity fractionation of lymphocytes using glass or plastic bead columns, *Scand. J. Immunol.* **5**(*Suppl.* 5): 23–29.

Wigzell, H., and Andersson, B., 1969, Cell separation on antigen coated columns. Elimination of high rate antibody forming cells and immunological memory cells, *J. Exp. Med.* **129**:23–24.

Wigzell, H., and Andersson, B., 1971, Isolation of lymphoid cells with active surface receptor sites, *Annu. Rev. Microbiol.* **25**:291–308.

Wigzell, H., and Mäkelä, O., 1970, Separation of normal and immune lymphoid cells by antigen-coated columns. Antigen-binding characteristics of membrane antibodies as analyzed by hapten-protein antigens, *J. Exp. Med.* **132**:110–125.

Wigzell, H., Sundquist, K. G., and Yoshida, T. O., 1972, Separation of cells according to surface antigens by the use of antibody-coated columns. Fractionation of cells carrying immunoglobulins and blood group antigen, *Scand. J. Immunol.* **1**:75–81.

Wilson, D. B., 1965, Quantitative studies on the behavior of sensitized lymphocytes *in vitro, J. Exp. Med.* **122**:143–152.

Wilson, J. D., 1973, The functions of immune T and B rosette-forming cells. *Immunology* **25**:185–191.

Winchester, R. J., and Ross, G., 1976, Methods for enumerating lymphocyte population, in *Manual of Clinical Immunology* (N. R. Rose and H. Friedman, eds.), pp. 64–76, American Society for Microbiology, Washington D.C.

Winchester, R. J., Fu, S. M., Hoffman, T., and Kunkel, H. G., 1975, IgG on lymphocyte surfaces: Technical problems and the significance of a third cell population, *J. Immunol.* **114**:1210–1214.

Wofsy, L., Kimura, J., and Truffa-Bachi, P., 1971, Cell separation on affinity columns: The preparation of pure populations of anti-hapten specific lymphocytes, *J. Immunol.* **107**:725–731.

Wybran, J., and Fudenberg, H. H., 1971, Rosette-formation, a test for cellular immunity. *Trans. Assoc. Am. Physicians* **84**:239–244.

Wybran, J., and Fudenberg, H. H., 1973, Thymus-derived rosette forming cells in various human disease states: cancer, lymphoma, bacterial and viral infections, and other diseases, *J. Clin. Invest.* **52**:1026–1032.

Wybran, J., Carr, M. C., and Fudenberg, H. H., 1972, The human rosette-forming cell as a marker of a population of thymus-derived cells, *J. Clin. Invest.* **51**:2537–2543.

Wybran, J., Carr, M. C., and Fudenberg, H. H., 1974, Effect of serum on human rosette forming cells in fetuses and adult blood, *Clin. Immunol. Immunopathol.* **1**:408–412.

Yefenof, E., Bakaes, T., Einham, L., Emberg, L., and Klein, G., 1978, Epstein-Barr virus (EBV) receptors, complement receptors, and EBV infectibility of different lymphocyte fractions of human peripheral blood. I. Complement receptor distribution and complement binding by separated lymphocyte subpopulations, *Cell. Immunol.* **35**:34–42.

Yodoi, J., Miyama, M., and Masuda, T., 1978, Immunological properties of Fc receptor on lymphocytes. 2. Differentiation from FcR− to FcR+ cells and their functional differences in *in vitro* antibody response, *Cell Immunol.* **35**:266–278.

Yoshida, T. O., and Andersson, B., 1972, Evidence for a receptor recognizing antigen complexed immunoglobulin on the surface of activated mouse thymus lymphocytes, *Scand. J. Immunol.* **1**:401–409.

Yu, D. T. Y. (1975) Human lymphocyte subpopulations: Early and late rosettes, *J. Immunol.* **115**:91–93.

Yu, D. T. Y., and Gale, R. P., 1977, Human lymphocyte subpopulations: Rabbit red blood cell rosettes, *J. Immunol. Methods* **16**:283–289.

Zighelboim, J., Gale, R. P., Chin, A., Bonavida, B., Ossorio, R. C., and Farey, J. L., 1974, Antibody dependent cellular cytotoxicity: Cytotoxicity mediated by non-T lymphocytes, *Clin. Immunol. Immunopathol.* **3**:193–198.

Zola, H., 1977, Fractionation of human lymphocytes using rosette formation with papain treated mouse erythrocytes, *J. Immunol. Methods* **18**:387–390.

Zoschke, D. C., and Bach, F. H., 1970, Specificity of antigen recognition by human lymphocytes *in vitro, Science* **170**:1404–1406.

Zoschke, D. C., and Bach, F. H., 1971a, *In vitro* elimination of specific immunoreactive cells with 5-bromodeoxyuridine, *J. Immunol. Methods* **1**:55–63.

Zoschke, D. C., and Bach, F. H., 1971b, Specificity of allogeneic cell recognition by human lymphocytes *in vitro, Science* **171**:1350–1352.

Index